P9-BIJ-382

Praise for *Dimming the Day*

"Jennifer Grant's *Dimming the Day* is a gift to an anxious world. From dandelions and redwoods to ginkgos and beehives, Grant uses the natural world as a springboard for spiritual insights. Keep this lovely book on your bedside table for reassurance and inspiration."

—Lori Erickson, author of *Near the Exit* and *Holy Rover*

"In *Dimming the Day*, Grant invites us to view the world through eyes of wonder. It is as if a kind friend has offered to tuck us in for the night, guiding us into glorious sleep."

—Shemaiah Gonzalez, writer

"Grant writes beautifully in a way that only someone who lives beautifully can do. This book is a rare antidote to the anxiety of our age."

—Jon M. Sweeney, author of *Feed the Wolf: Befriending Our Fears in the Way of Saint Francis*

"Jennifer Grant's reflections on creature and place in this bedtime companion intentionally settle the reader. It's an invitation to lay aside life's hustle and bustle and turn to a time of rest. Don't be surprised, though, if whimsical butterflies, dandelions, hummingbirds, and such enter your dreams."

—Traci Rhoades, author of *Not All Who Wander (Spiritually) Are Lost: A Story of Church*

"This gently penned, innovative collection of twenty evening meditations is an invitation to worry less about tomorrow and wonder more about the beauty of this earth and the great God who made it, in whose arms we can safely and securely fall asleep. *Dimming the Day* is destined to find a place on many a bedside table, including mine."

—Glenys Nellist, children's author of the Love Letters from God, Snuggle Time, and Little Mole series

"Into this chaotic and anxious world, *Dimming the Day* shows up as a soothing balm. Every word of this book has planted seeds for healing in my own weary heart, and I know it will do the same for others."

—April Fiet, author of *The Sacred Pulse: Holy Rhythms for Overwhelmed Souls*

"Exploring with obvious affection a marvelous breadth of created beings and creative artists, Grant has produced a piece that will induce both wonder and peace, inspiration, and calm. *Dimming the Day* is a book I can imagine keeping close at hand, to return to time and again."

—Rosalind C. Hughes, author of *A Family Like Mine: Biblical Stories of Love, Loss, and Longing* and *Whom Shall I Fear? Urgent Questions for Christians in an Age of Violence*

"A flood of adrenaline-sparking bad news coming at us through our screens shouts most of us to sleep each night. Jennifer Grant offers us an alternative in this book of wonder-filled reflections and grace-filled practices designed to gentle our souls as each day draws to a close."

—Michelle Van Loon, author of *Becoming Sage: Cultivating Maturity, Purpose, and Spirituality in Midlife*

"Author Jennifer Grant has an idea: Could we quiet our anxious thoughts by ending each day with awe and wonder? Weaving together nature, literature, faith, and daily life, Grant has produced a book of meditations and bedtime stories well worth keeping on your nightstand."

—Catherine McNiel, author of *All Shall Be Well: Awakening to God's Presence in His Messy, Abundant World*

"What an amazing, whimsical, informative, calming book! Although it's meant for an end-of-day read, it's perfect for any time you want to feel part of nature and centered. I'll be buying copies for family and friends."

—Dale Hanson Bourke, author of *Embracing Your Second Calling*

"*Dimming the Day* is an enchanting book by the immensely talented Jennifer Grant, who has the heart and soul of a poet. This is a book to savor, to muse upon, and to smile about as you drift off to sleep, dreaming of misty redwood groves, magical whale songs, and other deep and beautiful mysteries of our universe."

—Susy Flory, *New York Times* bestselling author or coauthor of 16 books, and director of West Coast Christian Writers

"In chapter after lovely chapter, Grant leads readers throughout the natural world, pointing out wondrous things and deftly connecting them to spiritual thoughts and practices before guiding us home and to rest. *Dimming the Day* is the perfect nightly companion for these wearying and perilous times."

—Alison Hodgson, author of *The Pug List: A Ridiculous Dog, a Family Who Lost Everything, and How They All Found Their Way Home*

"So many of us crawl into bed at night with our thoughts scrolling as fast as our news feeds. No wonder sleep eludes us. Jennifer Grant invites us to do things differently. A delicious blend of science and spirituality, this collection of reflections gently directs our gaze toward the marvelous complexity of the natural world. *Dimming the Day* is not only good for individual readers; it is good for our world."

—Laura Alary, author of *Breathe: A Child's Guide to Ascension, Pentecost, and the Growing Time*

"This small book goes deep and wide. Grant's soulful reflections and calming practices immerse us in the wild and winsome wonders of nature—a forest of mangroves, a murmuration of starlings, a solid ginkgo tree—to center our spirits before bed in a loving world and a loving God."

—Heidi Haverkamp, Episcopal priest and author of *Holy Solitude: Lenten Reflections with Saints, Hermits, Prophets, and Rebels*

"This book was a much-needed soul gift during a very difficult season. As each day dimmed, I found myself looking forward to the bright light of Grant's words and the stories in these pages."

—Rev. Tracey Bianchi, preaching pastor and adjunct seminary faculty

"In *Dimming the Day*, Jennifer Grant reminds me that to mark time by the sunset rather than my smartphone is to synchronize my spirit with the pulse of awe and wonder that beats at the heart of all creation."

—Milton Brasher-Cunningham, author of *The Color of Together: Mixed Metaphors of Connectedness*

"As someone who's struggled my entire life with sleep (and now has children who struggle too), *Dimming the Day* is what I've needed in ending the day with reassurance, gratitude, and awareness of God's presence as close as breath. I experienced Grant's beautiful stories and images as a calming, holy hug from the miraculous world itself, finding healing for my anxious heart and hope for my fragile soul. I will never look into the eyes of my child or taste honey or hear a red-winged blackbird the same way again."

—Rev. Arianne Braithwaite Lehn, author of *Ash and Starlight: Prayers for the Chaos and Grace of Daily Life*

DIMMING THE DAY

DIMMING THE DAY

EVENING MEDITATIONS FOR QUIET WONDER

JENNIFER GRANT

BROADLEAF BOOKS
MINNEAPOLIS

DIMMING THE DAY
Evening Meditations for Quiet Wonder

Copyright © 2021 Jennifer Grant. Printed by Broadleaf Books, an imprint of 1517 Media. All rights reserved. Except for brief quotations in critical articles or reviews, no part of this book may be reproduced in any manner without prior written permission from the publisher. Email copyright@1517.media or write to Permissions, Broadleaf Books, PO Box 1209, Minneapolis, MN 55440-1209.

Antonio Machado, "Last Night, as I Was Sleeping," in *Times Alone: Selected Poems of Antonio Machado*. Translation © 1983 by Robert Bly. Published by Wesleyan University Press and reprinted with permission.

Material excerpted from *The Showings of Julian of Norwich* © 2013 by Mirabai Starr used with permission from Hampton Roads Publishing c/o Red Wheel Weiser, LLC, Newburyport, MA (www.redwheelweiser.com).

Material excerpted from *The Inner Christ* © 1987 by John Main used with permission from Darton, Longman & Todd publishers, London, UK.

The prayer at the end of chapter 19 that begins "Holy God, your mercy is over all your works" is reprinted with permission. Published in the Episcopal Church's *Book of Occasional Services* © 2018 Church Publishing, New York, NY.

All Scripture quotations, unless otherwise indicated, are from the New Revised Standard Version Bible, copyright © 1989 the Division of Christian Education of the National Council of the Churches of Christ in the United States of America. Used by permission. All rights reserved.

Scripture quotations marked (KJV) are from the King James Version.

Scripture quotations marked (MSG) are taken from THE MESSAGE, copyright © 1993, 2002, 2018 by Eugene H. Peterson. Used by permission of NavPress, represented by Tyndale House Publishers. All rights reserved.

Scripture texts marked (NABRE) are taken from the *New American Bible, revised edition* © 2010, 1991, 1986, 1970 Confraternity of Christian Doctrine, Washington, D.C. and are used by permission of the copyright owner. All Rights Reserved. No part of the New American Bible may be reproduced in any form without permission in writing from the copyright owner.

Scripture quotations marked (NLT) are taken from the Holy Bible, New Living Translation, copyright ©1996, 2004, 2015 by Tyndale House Foundation. Used by permission of Tyndale House Publishers, Carol Stream, Illinois 60188. All rights reserved.

Cover design: Faceout Studios
Illustrations: Amanda Hudson

Print ISBN: 978-1-5064-7119-8
eBook ISBN: 978-1-5064-7120-4

Printed in Canada

For Astrid,
with love

Love all God's creation, the whole and every grain of sand in it. Love every leaf, every ray of God's light. Love the animals, love the plants, love everything. If you love everything, you will perceive the divine mystery in things. Once you perceive it, you will begin to comprehend it better every day. And you will come at last to love the whole world with an all-embracing love.

—Fyodor Dostoyevsky, *The Brothers Karamazov*

CONTENTS

INTRODUCTION

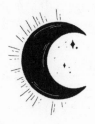

Sometimes anxiety is a restless toddler, overtired and squirming in your lap. Knocking up against you, it grips your shoulders with tiny fists. You try to speak calmly to it, but there's no reasoning with anxiety. You shift its weight; your arms ache from carrying it for so long. Rocking, you try to soothe it, try to help it relax. You want to ease it into sleep. *You* want to sleep.

But being in anxiety's clutches and getting a good night's sleep aren't compatible: it's one or the other. And many of us spend many unhappy nights in anxiety's company. While we toss and turn in bed, disappointments, mistakes, and failures play over and over in our minds. The future is full of uncertainty, and we catalog everything that could possibly go wrong in our lives and in the wider world. Doom scrolling through headlines in the middle of the night, we bear witness to hatred, inequality, and environmental ruin. And just when things seem to be calming down or improving, our world is shaken up again. It's like we're living in a snow globe, a storm of sorrow and injustice ever swirling around us. We're holding on by a thread.

I woke up yesterday to a short text one of my closest friends had written during the night. The time stamp was 2:50 a.m.:

"Can't sleep. Everything feels so broken."

THE AGE OF ANXIETY

So many of us are affected by mild to severe anxiety that it's now considered a normal part of human experience. A quick online search of the word *anxiety* results in descriptions of its "main types," including panic disorders and social or separation anxiety. It also suggests an endless assortment of ways to numb, treat, or escape it. Deep breathing. Meditation. Therapy. Antidepressants. Exercise. Cannabis oil. Counting to ten.

Psychologists differentiate between "normal anxiety," which is temporary and is often the response to a specific situation, and "clinically relevant anxiety disorders," which can be disabling, persist over time, and significantly disrupt a person's life. If you wonder whether your anxiety is normal or clinically relevant, I encourage you to speak to a doctor or therapist and to visit adaa.org, the website for the Anxiety and Depression Association of America. When I talk about anxiety in this book, I'm referring to normal anxiety, which can be agonizing to suffer from but is impermanent. Normal anxiety can be at least somewhat alleviated by moving our bodies, eating healthy food, breathing deeply, connecting with others—and, yes, getting enough sleep.

An article written in 2018 gives this current period in the United States and the United Kingdom the nickname "the age of anxiety," noting, "It would be bizarre if most of us . . . weren't anxious: inequality is skyrocketing, the job market is becoming more precarious and house prices are increasingly out of reach. Add in political instability and there is a lot to worry about. The one thing you shouldn't worry about, however, is that you are the only one feeling anxious."

And that was written two years *before* the COVID-19 pandemic.

Although those of us who were raised in the church were taught from a very young age not to "worry about tomorrow" (see Matthew 6:34), people of faith ruminate on the past and worry about the future just like everybody else. We end the day by swiping through our newsfeeds on social media just like everybody else does. We're anxious . . . just like everybody else.

So how might people living in the age of anxiety respond to the Divine invitation not to worry about the past or the future but instead to live in the present moment? Maybe one way is to end each day differently.

Dimming the Day isn't about glossing over or denying the trouble we are or the world is in. It's not about numbing our pain or looking away from suffering and injustice. It's not an upbeat reminder to practice self-care. Instead, this book is an invitation to connect with something deep and true at the end of the day. You could consider it a gentle tap on your shoulder prompting you to turn away from the blue light of your device so that your mind can be calmed and you can get a good night's sleep.

But *how?*

THE BENEFITS OF AWE

Let's return to that restless toddler—Anxiety—who was squirming in your lap. Imagine for a moment that you and Anxiety are sitting beside an open window and a monarch butterfly glides into the room, catching your attention. There's a vase of cut wildflowers on the sill, and the butterfly flits around it before landing on a pale pink milkweed bloom. The steady motion of its black and orange wings as they open and close is mesmerizing. Anxiety's shoulders drop, and its mouth opens in awe. Seeing something beautiful—actually experiencing a sense of *wonder*—has soothed Anxiety. It lets out a deep sigh and, finally, relaxes in your arms.

I learned about this surprising fringe benefit to experiencing awe a couple of years ago when, while reading up on positive psychology for a writing assignment, I happened on a series of videos produced by the Greater Good Science Center (GGSC), based at the University of California, Berkeley. GGSC "studies the psychology, sociology, and neuroscience of well-being and teaches skills that foster a thriving, resilient, and compassionate society."

One of the videos features researcher Craig Anderson, who says that experiencing awe is a powerful and effective antidote to anxiety. Anderson writes, "Awe happens when you encounter something so vast that you don't feel like you wrap your mind around it completely, right at that moment. So, awe could involve experiences of profound beauty, or feeling super-connected to other people or to nature or to humanity as a whole."

Experiencing wonder and awe, he and others in his field have claimed, alters the way we understand the world. Awe promotes *pro*social—as opposed to *anti*social—behavior, stimulating positive actions such as helping or comforting others. It also relieves stress. Even watching videos or looking at pictures of natural beauty can have a positive effect on our brains; some have called such images "visual valium." Additionally, one of Anderson's studies showed that when people with mental health disorders experienced awe in nature, some subjects—even ones suffering from post-traumatic stress disorder (PTSD)—actually *recovered* their mental health.

Experiencing awe has still other benefits to our health and well-being. Studies show that feeling awe or wonder reduces inflammation, helps us think more critically, decreases materialism, and expands our perception of time, making us feel more "time rich." And, yes, it has been shown to help us sleep better.

Awe also affects us spiritually. In a study published in the *Journal for the Study of Religion, Nature and Culture*, researchers found that children who regularly play outside in nature have a higher appreciation for beauty and a heightened sense of wonder and awe than children who do not. The children in the study expressed feelings of "peacefulness" and a calm sense of belonging. They felt more alive and connected to the world than did their peers. They felt aware of a higher power, a "divine sense or mystery."

That resonates with me. Over the years, when my church has gathered outdoors at a park or forest preserve for Eucharist in the summertime, I've felt more aware of the presence of the Divine than almost any experience I can remember having *within* the walls of a church. The warm rays of sunshine feel like God's love shining down. The clouds seem to hover near us, hoping to catch a strain of our song. Canada geese, honking as they come in for a landing on the surface of the lake, are like latecomers to the service, quarreling over whose fault it is that they missed the opening bell. The clover and grass under my feet feel more familiar and comforting than the embroidered kneelers at church. I feel humbled on those summer Sunday mornings, more aware of how small I am and, at the same time, how good it is to be a person, alive and out in the world.

URGENT BIOPHILIA

I'm writing this in 2020, a year of dramatic revisions, reckonings, and revelations. In January, no one could have imagined how much "normal" life was about to change. We couldn't have begun to grasp how our perspectives would radically shift, in very short order. Many of us began to see with new eyes the unjust systems, institutions, and assumptions that have been foundational to our way of life. Forced to slow down to a crawl, we have taken a good hard look at what we consume and the way our behavior has affected the health of the planet. We've seen ourselves, our choices, and our society up close and more precisely than ever before. It's been a magnifying glass of a time, humbling, wearying, and hard. The burden of loss on both the personal and the global levels has been divided and distributed. Some people carry a much larger portion of it than others, but everyone, to some extent, bears it. Of course this affects our ability to rest.

A friend tells me about his recent sleep issues. He falls asleep around ten o'clock, wakes at midnight, and lies awake for the rest of the night, stumbling out of bed at six or seven o'clock to start the coffee and make breakfast for his children. Another friend says the only way she can find her way to sleep is to play a round of golf, mentally, hole by hole, until she drifts off. Another says the way he self-soothes in the night is to imagine he's in a darkened room looking at tropical fish swimming around inside an aquarium. In the middle of the night, I've done everything from playing rain sounds on my phone to listening to a meditation app to staring out the window for hours, keeping watch over the empty street.

As political tensions rise, businesses fumble and fail, educators and parents and community leaders hustle to adapt to new realities, and the human community in general, across the globe, continues to wrestle with what life looks and feels like now, one thing has been a source of surprise and happiness for me. It's the way many of us have changed our relationship with nature during the pandemic. Mine has deepened, to be sure.

I've lived in the same house for fifteen years and have walked through the park at the end of my street countless times. But when the country shut down, my family and I began taking daily walks together. In March, we walked in the snow and biting wind. We walked in April's rain as the buds on the trees began to swell. We walked in May, with the bushes and flowers in celebratory bloom. We walked in the heat of July and August, the grass scorched and brown beneath our feet. Now the chill is back in the air; I grab a coat as we head out the back gate. Yesterday afternoon, snow swirled around us on our walk.

The park has been a part of my life as long as I've lived here, but I have a new relationship with it. Bearing witness every single day to the trees and wildflowers and birds, I watch the seasons change as if in slow motion. Winter turns to spring and spring to summer and summer to fall and now fall to winter again. I've come to see this place with brand-new eyes. I'm reminded of G. K. Chesterton's promise: "If you look at a thing nine hundred and ninety-nine times, you are perfectly safe; if you look at it the thousandth time, you are in frightful danger of seeing it for the first time." During lockdown, I've seen my neighborhood park for the thousandth time and, in some ways, for the very first time. It has been a gift.

I've come to recognize—or, if you're in a more pragmatic mood, you could argue, *impose*—distinct personalities on the trees and birds and wildlife there. Previously, they just sort of made up the general elements of "the park" in my mind. But now, waving at me from across the field, the white poplars seem playful and welcoming. Their leaves are green on one side, silver on the other, like a child's sequined sweatshirt, the spangles flipping to reveal a hidden design. The way their bark is bedazzled by the diamond pattern of their air pores makes them even flashier. Red-winged blackbirds, their red and yellow feathers like fancy epaulets on a military uniform, usually stay back from the path, hidden in the reeds near the water. A few months ago, they hissed at us and went on the attack, warning us to keep our distance from their nests. The line of four turtles who watch us, utterly still from their log in the lake, seem bemused at our determined strides. "What's the hurry?" they seem to ask.

That it feels *good* to be outside makes sense; we're actually hardwired to want to connect with nature. Erich Fromm invented the word *biophilia* to describe this, defining it as "the passionate love of life and of all that is alive." That desire to connect with all that is alive during this time has people all over the globe going out on walks, clearing out animal shelters to bring home new creaturely companions, and planting gardens like they never have before. In a recent magazine article, published several months into the pandemic, journalist Rebecca Mead explores the benefits of gardening to mental health. She quotes a therapist in that piece as saying, "Whenever there's a crisis—be it a war, or the aftermath of war, or a natural disaster—we see this phenomenon of urgent biophilia. . . . We gain sustenance from nature's regeneration."

DIMMING THE DAY

Being outside—or even looking at photos and watching videos of natural beauty—soothes us, as does experiencing wonder and awe in our imaginations as we contemplate the natural world. This book is an invitation for you to end your day by powering off your devices and redirecting your gaze, inwardly at least, toward nature. I invite you to calm that restless toddler who's been squirming in your lap and to replace the worries in your mind with a sense of awe. After you get into bed, take a few moments to sit or lie quietly, and just become aware that you are sitting or lying still. Take a few deep breaths, and signal to your body that you are done for the day and ready to wind down. Then dim your day by reading part of this book.

Each of its twenty chapters focuses on one subject or place and includes reflections by poets, mystics, theologians, novelists, and others whose words give voice to our shared biophilia—or love for all that is alive—in fresh ways. Each chapter contains a relaxation exercise or prayer to help you settle down for a peaceful night's sleep. Use the prompts for sleep in whatever way works best for you. Perhaps a phrase from a poem will stand out to you as you read it. Hold on to those words, perhaps using them as a mantra, repeating them silently after you've turned out the lights and are drifting off to sleep.

To be clear, this isn't a science textbook but rather reflections on nature to bring calm at the end of the day. One of the many writers whose words I share here is American conservationist John Burroughs. You might not yet know his work but have probably heard his famous advice: "Leap and the net will appear!" Like me, Burroughs regarded himself not as a scientist but as a person who loved to write about his relationship with, and appreciation for, the natural world. He wrote that he didn't coldly study nature but "visited with her." He said these visits soothed and healed him and put his senses "in tune once more." The reflections in this book are meant to put the senses in tune at the end of the day.

As it's a book to be read at bedtime, you might be wondering, What if I fall asleep while reading a chapter? Well then, my friend, I've done my job! At the back of this book, I've included my favorite prayer for bedtime, from the Book of Common Prayer. You could return to it night after night if you like, just before sleep, or mark that page and open to it if you find yourself awake in the night. It begins, "Keep watch, dear Lord, with those who work, or watch, or weep this night." This prayer has given me words more times than I can count—times when my mind and my heart are full, but I don't know what to say.

While I can't take you on a walk through the redwoods or pluck you a dandelion from the sidewalk, and while we can't sit side by side and look up at the night sky tonight, we can consider these things together, these lovely things, and end the day in quiet wonder.

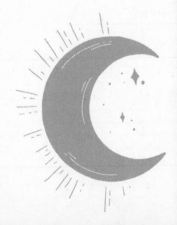

I
EYES
A HUNDRED UNIVERSES

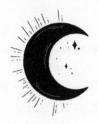

Reading fine print was never a problem for me until—all of a sudden—it was. So dramatic was the decline that I made an appointment with a doctor. When she came into the exam room, I blurted out that something was very wrong. The doctor looked up from her clipboard. My voice shook as I described how abruptly my vision had changed.

"How old are you?" she asked.

When I said I'd turned forty the week before, she actually laughed at me.

"You're fine," she said. "You're just getting old."

She then launched into an explanation of how aging affects eyesight, how, in the human eye, the lens becomes less flexible, less adept at focusing on things up close as we get older. By age fifty, she assured me, nearly everybody experiences this.

It seems just as common that as we get older, we stop seeing what's right in front of us in a figurative sense as well. The lenses through which we perceive the world are at risk of getting as inflexible as the ones in our eyes. We stop looking at the people and world around us with curiosity. No longer fueled by the wonder we felt when we were younger, we start to skim over what has become most familiar to us. But neuroscientists insist there *are* ways to train our brains to be more flexible, more alert, and more aware. One way is to pay close attention to the present moment.

Mindful seeing is a meditation practice that slows our thoughts and takes us to a place where we are simply noticing something, right where we are. There's not a right way or wrong way to practice mindful seeing—just focus your gaze on one thing and notice everything about it: shapes, colors, and lines.

Sitting in bed, I look across the room to the piece of art hanging on the wall opposite me. I bought it more than twenty-five years ago in Hanoi, Vietnam. The gallery where I found it, down a tiny lane in the Old Quarter of the city, was one of several galleries there, all in a row. It's an outdoor scene drawn in colorful oil pastels on burlap. A huge orange sun shines down on two water buffalo. There are three human figures in the picture: a man riding a water buffalo, another reclining on one, and a woman kneeling on the ground, shading herself with an iconic, conical hat. Done in a Cubist style, the artwork communicates a sense of calm and drew me in from the start. I've had it for so long that I realized recently that I've stopped really *seeing* it. I've stopped being charmed by its bright colors and its peaceful tableau. I've been skimming past it, hardly giving it a glance.

To look at this drawing mindfully doesn't involve calling to mind the memory of purchasing it or dissecting the elements of what makes it Cubist or otherwise a compelling piece of art. It's not about *thinking* but about simply *seeing*. To look at the drawing mindfully, I focus on it and notice the shapes and colors. The round orange sun. The green jumble of trees in the background. Hats, two yellow triangles. Black spirals. It's not about art appreciation or judging things as good or bad. Mindful seeing is just about being aware of what you are looking at, right where you are. It feels good to see this work again, to let its shapes and colors wash over me.

Marcel Proust is often quoted—on mugs, wall hangings, and memes—as saying, "The real voyage of discovery consists, not in seeking new landscapes, but in having new eyes." That's a nice thought, to be sure, but the actual quote is more complicated and beautiful than that. In his novel

In Search of Lost Time, Proust writes, "The only true voyage of discovery, the only fountain of Eternal Youth, would be not to visit strange lands but to possess other eyes, to behold the universe through the eyes of another, of a hundred others, to behold the hundred universes that each of them beholds, that each of them is."

Awe is the underlying theme of this book. Essentially, though, it's a book about *seeing*, so we begin by looking at the wonder of the human eye. The eye *is* a marvel, not only in its design and function, but because of what it can tell us about the "hundred universes" inside of every single one of us.

After the brain, the eye is the most complex organ in the human body. It contains 130 million light-sensitive cells called cones and rods. In case you need a refresher from biology class, the cones detect color (and the human eye can see about ten million different variations), while the rods, highly responsive to low-intensity light, allow us to see at nighttime. When light reflects off objects and enters the human eye, we see. The cornea is the clear outer layer at the front of the eye and helps the eye focus light. The cornea has the highest concentration of nerve endings in the body, hundreds of times greater than the skin. The iris, that colored tissue also at the front of the eye, is a muscle. Both its color and its textural patterns—ridges and folds—are as unique to a person as a fingerprint. Actually, it's even *more* unique: a fingerprint has 40 distinct traits, while the iris has

240 or more. Even one person's two irises aren't identical; each and every iris is one of a kind.

The muscles in the eye are the most active and fastest muscles in the body. Even when we're staring at something, our eyes are at work moving around and creating a mental three-dimensional map of what we see. These quick, jerky eye movements are called saccades; occurring several times a second, they're quicker than a heartbeat. And we don't even notice them!

The pupil is a hole at the center of the iris protected by the cornea, and it controls how much light enters the eye. And more than fulfilling that important function, it reveals much about a person's emotional state. "Pupillary response" describes how pupils shrink in bright light and expand in the dark. But pupils adjust in size in response not only to the brightness of the environment but also to the amount of light a person *expects* to encounter. Pupils dilate when a person is provoked by a threat or an opportunity; they respond when we are aroused, whether by sexual attraction or a problem that we wish to puzzle out, or when we are listening well to someone else. Irene Loewenfeld, a pioneer of pupillometry, or the measurement of pupil size and response, said, "Man may either blush or turn pale . . . but his pupils always dilate." Our eyes truly are windows into our souls.

Our eyes also offer glimpses into the state of our general physical health. An eye exam can detect many health problems, including high blood pressure and thyroid disease. Damage to blood vessels in the retina can point to diabetes. Inflammation in the optic nerves can signal multiple sclerosis . . . and the list goes on.

Our eyes are windows into our pasts too. A university research study published in 2020 found that the eyes of people with PTSD react differently to stimuli than those who haven't experienced severe trauma. The pupils of patients with PTSD have an exaggerated response when viewing exciting or dangerous images—whether they are violent images or positive scenes, such as thrilling athletic victories.

Some therapists say the eyes can also be the key to *processing* past trauma. In the 1980s, a psychologist invented a therapeutic technique called eye movement desensitization and reprocessing (EMDR) after discovering that moving her eyes from side to side helped her deal with painful memories. In EMDR therapy, a patient identifies an unpleasant or painful memory and then, with the help of a trained clinician, is led through gentle, deliberate eye movements. EMDR involves "bringing distressing trauma-related images, beliefs, and bodily sensations to mind, whilst the therapist guides eye movements from side to side. More positive views of the trauma memories are identified, with the aim of replacing the distressing ones." So our eyes can not only *reveal* excitement or a sense of well-being or fear; they can also help *heal* us from memories that cause suffering.

This discussion of the human eye would be incomplete without at least a brief look at tears. Again, they are more intricate than, well, meets the eye. Did you know that glands around the eyes actually produce *three* distinct types of tears?

Basal tears are continuously released into the eye in very small amounts to lubricate the cornea, keeping it clear of dust and other matter. They also are part of the immune system, as they fight against bacterial infection.

Reflex tears also work to protect the eyes from outside irritants but are produced in larger amounts when our eyes are stung by vapors—like when you are chopping onions or get assaulted by a perfume ad in a glossy magazine. Reflex tears are also released when we cough or yawn.

Emotional or *psychic tears* are generated when we experience strong feelings. They contain stress hormones, so when we're having a good cry, we are actually relieving and releasing stress from our bodies. Emotional tears stabilize a person's mood quickly and stimulate the body to produce endorphins, feel-good hormones. A cleansing cry slows our breathing and releases stress. After it, we feel soothed.

In their book *Burnout: The Secret to Unlocking the Stress Cycle*, authors Emily Nagoski and Amelia Nagoski explain that in order to deal with stress effectively and prevent burnout, we need to "complete the stress response cycle," or, they say, "complete" our emotions. This means that after we've had a stressful experience (like having a particularly busy and frustrating week at work or having an argument with a friend), we need to signal to our bodies that we're safe and all is well again. This "completes" the stress response. If we don't do this, we can get stuck in negative feelings and, ultimately, become emotionally exhausted. The authors explain that in order to communicate with the body, we have to use *its* language. We can't just tell ourselves "OK, that's over now" to switch off the tangled, half-completed emotions we feel after a stressful experience. (Remember, you can't reason with toddlers *or* anxiety!)

To complete the stress response cycle, according to the Nagoskis, we must use language that our *bodies* understand, including deep breathing, exercise, and—you guessed it!—having what they call "A Big Ol' Cry" and releasing those emotional tears. Watch your favorite tearjerker movie, they recommend, noting, "Going through that emotion with the characters allows your body to go through it, too."

Our eyes are unique—the colors and textures of our irises are as distinct as snowflakes. They hold the clues not only to our physical health but to what inspires and arouses us. They reveal our character and the state of our soul. They produce tears to regulate and calm our emotions and help us recover from stress.

No wonder Jesus said in Luke 11:34 that when a person's eyes are healthy, their whole body is full of light.

◆

Read Proust's words again: "The only true voyage of discovery, the only fountain of Eternal Youth, would be not to visit strange lands but to possess other eyes, to behold the universe through the eyes of another, of a hundred others, to behold the hundred universes that each of them beholds, that each of them is."

◆

Close your eyes for a few moments, and then let them softly flutter open again.

Then take three slow, deep, cleansing breaths.

Now inhale deeply again, and as you exhale, let that out breath continue a few seconds longer than your inhale. (Try, for instance, breathing in for four seconds through your nose and out for eight through the mouth. This doesn't need to be exact: do whatever count feels calming and comfortable to you. Practice this a few times.)

Right now, right here, practice a few moments of a mindful seeing meditation. Look up from this book at something in the space around you. Focus on something you've stopped really seeing. Notice colors and textures. Don't judge what you're seeing as good or bad or as beautiful or ugly or as special or commonplace.

Don't tell a story about it. Just notice what's there, right where you are. Accept whatever it is, just as it is. Try to see it with fresh eyes.

As you drift off to sleep, remember that the eyes with which you see the world are uniquely yours.

No one else has irises just the same color or pattern as yours.

No one else has seen what you have seen.

No one else has cried the tears that you have cried.

Tonight, look with kindness on the hundred universes that you are.

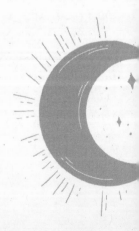

2

DANDELIONS

THE MIRACULOUS IN THE COMMON

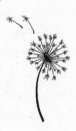

The groundskeepers have just mowed the park. Walking across the meadow, I kick at thick, matted clumps of grass. Then I spy, a few feet ahead of me, a lone dandelion standing up straight. About six or seven inches tall, its puff of silver seeds is a perfect globe. I wonder how it remained untouched: Did it somehow duck down, protecting its mane, until the mower passed? I bend down and pluck it, and its hollow stem makes a soft pop. I look at its seeds; they're tiny parachutes waiting for release. I inhale deeply and then, like a child making a wish, release my breath and watch the seeds take flight.

When my children were little, I discouraged them from blowing dandelion seeds. Instead, I paid them a nickel or dime for every yellow head they snapped off the plants in early spring. It was my inexpensive, eco-friendly attempt at weed control, and it worked fairly well. But I see dandelions differently now. If I could do it all over again, I'd invite my kids to blow the seeds like a million wishes into the breeze whenever they found a dandelion that had gone to seed.

All those years ago, I didn't know that dandelions are a key food source for pollinators. Bees, butterflies, and moths—like the whimsically named "pearl-bordered fritillary," named for the row of pearly markings along the underedges of its wings—love them. Songbirds including white-throated sparrows, American goldfinches, and indigo buntings feast on dandelion seeds too.

As a young mother and new homeowner in a pristine suburb, I thought a lawn full of dandelions was cause for shame. Dandelions were noxious: unwelcome weeds and nothing more.

But it wasn't always this way. Dandelions have been a key element in traditional Chinese medicine for millennia and were prized by ancient Egyptians, Romans, and Greeks in their pharmacies as well. Dandelions can be used to treat infections and to address other medical problems, like heartburn, constipation, and liver disorders. In Victorian England, they were considered a delicacy and served in salads and sandwiches.

Dandelions came to North America with the English in the seventeenth century. They brought seeds from home and planted and tended the plants. The frugal Puritans loved them, as every part of the plant can be eaten—its root, stem, and flower. Rich in vitamins A, C, and K and high in calcium, iron, magnesium, and potassium, they're nutritious too. Their yellow flowers are also used to make natural dyes. Dandelion flowers are still used to make wine, and some breweries today use the greens as a substitute for hops. No wonder that for so long, they were a fixture in kitchen gardens.

Before the nineteenth century in North America, land around both Indigenous peoples' and colonists' homes was used for vegetable and herb gardens and for animals to graze. Only after Thomas Jefferson created manicured gardens at Monticello did surrounding one's home with a perfect, weedless lawn come into fashion in the dominant culture. Fast-forward to today, when Americans spend millions of dollars a year on lawn pesticides to maintain uniform lawns of nonnative grasses, using 30 percent of the country's water supply to keep them lush and green.

So despite the good work the modest dandelion does for insects, people, and even other plants—their deep and sturdy taproots bring nutrients closer to the ground, helping nearby shallow-rooted plants—they have been banished from our properties.

After I blow the seeds away, I notice a drop of milky liquid on my hand. The sap that has spilled out of its stem is actually latex, containing natural rubber. Something like twenty thousand species of plants produce latex, but only a fraction of these contain rubber in their sap. Rubber, of course, is ever in high demand for making tires, toys, medical devices, shoes, and so much more. The fact that rubber can be produced from dandelion milk once again points to the value of this unassuming plant. Scientists in Germany and Belgium have developed technologies to make natural rubber from dandelions that is the same quality as that produced from rubber trees. (The plants and animals whose ecosystems are threatened by rubber plantations thank the dandelion most wholeheartedly.)

Food. Medicine. Tea. Dye. Wine. Beer. Latex. As if all of those contributions weren't enough, dandelions are also beautiful. Their yellow-orange flowers are actually made up of tiny individual flowers called "ray florets," and the bloom opens at sunrise and closes at night. And although you might think it's called dande*lion* because of that yellow mane, its name actually comes from the French *dent de lion*, meaning "tooth of the lion," for the jagged shape of its leaves.

Dandelions grow fast, their roots are deep, and they can survive harsh conditions. These traits have led psychologists to develop new metaphors to describe mental and emotional resilience, naming highly sensitive individuals "orchids," medium-sensitive people "tulips," and yes, low-sensitive folks "dandelions." Most of us, by the way, are tulips (40 percent), while 31 percent of us are orchids: individuals who are generally more sensitive or fragile, who do exceptionally well in ideal conditions and exceptionally badly in poor ones. About 29 percent of us are dandelions: resilient, generally less sensitive to the surrounding environment, and able to grow fairly well anywhere.

Walking up the driveway, back home again from the park, I look at the dandelion stem in my hand and wonder, How many times did I walk over one, fail to notice one, or otherwise miss the everyday miracle of this plant?

♦

The dandelion is the only flower that represents three celestial bodies during different phases of its life cycle—sun, moon, and stars. The yellow flower of the plant resembles the sun. The puffball, when it has gone to seed, looks like the moon. And the dispersing seeds of the plant are like stars. It is a miracle.

In his essay Nature, *Ralph Waldo Emerson describes the energy and joy human beings can derive from nature. He saw everything in the natural world as an "incarnation of God" and an "expositor of the divine mind." Emerson seems to have lived with a sense of urgent biophilia, ever delighting in the natural world and looking, with wonder, on what it reveals about the Divine.* Nature *begins,*

> *The lover of nature is he whose inward and outward senses are still truly adjusted to each other; who has retained*

the spirit of infancy even into the era of manhood. His intercourse with heaven and earth, becomes part of his daily food. In the presence of nature, a wild delight runs through the man, in spite of real sorrows. . . . Crossing a bare common, in snow puddles, at twilight, under a clouded sky, without having in my thoughts any occurrence of special good fortune, I have enjoyed a perfect exhilaration. I am glad to the brink of fear. In the woods too, a man casts off his years, as the snake his slough, and at what period soever of life, is always a child. In the woods, is perpetual youth. . . . A decorum and sanctity reign, a perennial festival is dressed, and the guest sees not how he should tire of them in a thousand years.

Emerson ended his essay with a sentence that crystallizes the content of the entire work, the oft quoted words "The invariable mark of wisdom is to see the miraculous in the common." Dandelions give us the opportunity to do just that.

♦

Close your eyes, take a deep breath in through your nose, and then let it out through your mouth before opening your eyes again.

With the delight of a child, imagine holding a dandelion that's gone to seed in your hand. Feel the stem between your fingertips. With your mind's eye, see the dandelion's silver globe of wishes.

Inhale deeply and gently blow over them, sending them out into the world. Imagine your wishes flying far, landing and finding soil, and sprouting into young green shoots.

Tonight, as you settle down, reflect on the miracle of your own life.

Consider that, like a dandelion, you are sometimes like the sun, sometimes like the moon, and sometimes like the stars.

Your presence adds value to the lives of those around you.

You bring healing, nourishment, and beauty into the world.

You are resilient and your roots grow deep.

What good things do you wish for yourself tonight?

For someone else?

For the world?

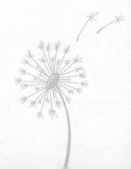

3
HUMPBACK WHALES

A MYSTICAL OUTCRYING

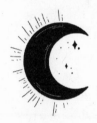

Old Fisherman's Wharf in Monterey, California, is a tourist destination with all the usual trappings: souvenir shops, "press a penny" machines, caricature artists, silver and crystal jewelry stands, and sweetshops where passersby can watch saltwater taffy and fudge being made. As a fishing town on the ocean, Monterey brags that it's the "former sardine capital of the world"; fish-and-chips shops and fine-dining seafood restaurants abound.

It's a historic place where—even before there was a city called Monterey—whales filled the bay. In the 1850s, whaling companies began operations there, hunting gray, humpback, and other whales primarily for their blubber. The blubber would be boiled and made into oil to fuel lamps, lubricate machinery, and produce soap and other goods.

The city has literary significance too. Three of John Steinbeck's most famous novels (*Tortilla Flat*, *Cannery Row*, and *Sweet Thursday*) are set in Monterey, and statues and plaques and other tributes celebrating him are scattered around the area. Steinbeck grew up nearby in Central California and was close friends with Ed Ricketts, an eccentric, brilliant marine biologist whose lab was steps away from Old Fisherman's Wharf.

In 1940, a year after *The Grapes of Wrath* was published, he and Ricketts sailed to the Sea of Cortez in Mexico, also known as the Gulf of California, to survey marine life. Steinbeck's life had been turned upside down by sudden wealth and fame after his novel won the Pulitzer Prize. Steinbeck was also receiving death threats: with its story of the injustices and suffering endured by migrant farmworkers, the book was being taken by some as a communist treatise or otherwise a threat to the status quo. Members of the Associated Farmers, a group of landowners who opposed organized labor, burned copies of the novel, and it was banned from libraries around the United States. This virulent criticism likely contributed to the author's desire to disappear for those six weeks with his friend.

After their trip, Steinbeck wrote *The Log from the Sea of Cortez*, a book that catalogs not only the sea creatures he and Ricketts observed but the people they met and their reflections on religion, happiness, and what it is to be human. In it, Steinbeck writes, "We ran from collecting station to new collecting station, and when the night came and the anchor was dropped, a quiet came over the boat. . . . And then we talked and speculated, talked and drank beer. And our discussion ranged from the loveliness of remembered women to the complexities of relationships."

Steinbeck later told his wife that he considered this work of nonfiction the very best book of his entire career. Part travelogue, part philosophy, it's full of awe-inspiring reflections on the interconnectedness of all of nature. Rickett's biographer said the biologist saw "everything as interrelated parts of the whole. . . . There was no difference between a good poem, an interesting piece of music, and . . . a sea spider."

My daughter and I are in Monterey for the day, on a weekend trip to visit my son in California. Whale watching is at the top of her wish list for our time here, and I am happy to comply. Pulling away from the dock on our tour, we hear the guttural, goofy barking of sea lions and the screeches of seagulls, and we watch sea otters gently backstroking through the water, some with their babies riding along on their chests. These creatures—not the busking street musicians or people hawking Monterey T-shirts or nautical decor from gift shops—are the true proprietors of the bay.

When you scan the horizon for signs of sea creatures, eager for a sighting, it's easy to be fooled into thinking the crest of a wave in the distance is actually a whale that has come up to the surface. But the tour guide has a keen eye and will announce, "Look over at ten o'clock" or "Pod of dolphins at three o'clock," interrupting herself from her lecture on the bay or about the migration patterns of whales. The boat is like the center of a clock face, with marine life and birds dancing around the hours.

A massive flock of seabirds called sooty shearwaters lands on the water, their call somehow a combination of a mourning dove's coo and the bray of a donkey. There are humpbacks below, the guide explains, and the seabirds are feeding off the fish and squid that the whales disturb or the scraps from their meals that float to the surface. Then, all of a sudden, a whale begins to breach, and the shearwaters fly off. The humpback's black body rises out of the water as though it's balanced on an elevated platform.

Nothing has prepared me for the enormity of this creature or how to take in its massive, elegant self. A moment later, it arches and dives down, waving goodbye with its perfect flukes. The birds return, and I wonder for a moment whether I've only imagined the whole thing.

Every year, the guide explains, after the whales disappear out of sight for the season, humpbacks' round-trip migration is thousands of miles as they travel from the California coast to warmer waters closer to the equator and back again. Biologists, like the ones in Monterey, can identify individual humpbacks from the scars and notches and white patches and other markings on their flukes. Some whales return to the same waters year after year. The guide speaks about some of them as though they are her old friends.

From the deck of the boat, the only sounds from the humpback that we can hear are the smack of its massive body hitting the surface of the water and the rush of air through its blowholes. But everyone on board knows that the male humpback loves to sing. His songs echo and carry for miles deep underwater. The female humpback makes noises too, but she doesn't sing what you could describe as organized songs.

But *why* do they sing? Traditionally, whale songs have been understood to be mating calls, but more recent research suggests that there is more nuance to this phenomenon than that. When males move somewhere new, they change their songs to match those that nearby whales are singing. But why? So they can fit into a new social group? So they won't seem like outsiders to the females in this new locale? To show dominance over other males?

Some researchers suggest that humpbacks learn new songs to help them better find their way on their journeys: they understand exactly where they are based on the distinctive songs whales in different locations sing. ("Ah . . . I hear 'The Yellow Rose of Texas,' so I must be near Galveston," a whale might think.)

Humpbacks' songs are actually distinctive to their own particular breeding grounds. When it's time to mate, humpbacks return to the exact location where they were born. Gathering there, the males sing a song that is, as one writer says, "common to that breeding ground, almost like it's a local jingle or a college fight song." And those songs evolve year after year; the whales add in or take out parts of the song, affected by what they've heard from other whales on their journeys. The farther apart their breeding grounds, the more different the humpbacks' songs are. Humpbacks born in the Indian Ocean, for example, sing songs that sound very different from ones who were born in the Pacific.

We didn't even know that humpback whales sang until the 1950s, when US military intelligence officers who were trying to hear transmissions from Russian submarines instead heard *them*. The fact that not too long ago, we knew *nothing* of their songs helps explain why we don't yet know, conclusively, why and how the humpback sings. But most researchers now agree that humpback culture is not only revealed but *transmitted* through their songs.

In his stunning book *Becoming Wild: How Animal Cultures Raise Families, Create Beauty, and Achieve Peace*, author Carl Safina writes that the male humpback whale's "strange and haunting singing is a changeable cultural aspect of his species. Each year, all adult male humpbacks within each ocean sing the same song. . . . And each year, the song of each ocean changes . . . all the whales adopting the same changed elements of the song."

Humpbacks aren't the only whales to sing, but their songs are the most elaborate. They are composed of moans, howls, and growling. And these songs are more organized, our guide explains, than they might initially seem. Like our own musical compositions, in humpback songs, a series of sounds is repeated in patterns over time; marine biologists (and human composers) call these "phrases." The repeated phrases, then, compose a theme, and there are five to seven themes in each humpback song. The sounds aren't made by vocal cords; humpback whales don't have them. Instead, they produce sounds by pushing air through chambers in their respiratory system. Their songs cover frequencies that cannot be heard by humans and can last up to twenty minutes long. While singing, the whale floats, nearly motionless.

You can listen to humpback songs online, although good luck trying to discern the phrases and themes of each song. What I hear is a wide range of sounds that seem both mechanical and somehow natural—low growls and high cries and whines. Some sounds are like the muted, restrained barking of a dreaming dog. Others are like someone running their fingernails up and down the strings of an acoustic guitar.

Then there's a kind of siren and the screech of a seagull. I hear a cow mooing, then the bellowing of a bull.

Whether they are trying to attract potential mates, establish dominance, find their way across the ocean, or just simply express themselves, the humpbacks' songs sound to me like lament. In the Hebrew Bible, a selection of seven psalms (Psalms 44, 60, 74, 79, 80, 85, and 90) are referred to as the "psalms of communal lament." These particular psalms express sorrow for a large body of people and the troubles of a nation and ask for God's blessing. Christians throughout history have used these psalms after a natural disaster, plague, or other tragedy.

During 2020, many faith communities held special services to make communal laments. We lamented the pandemic and the suffering and loss of life it has left in its wake. We lamented police brutality and systemic racism. We lamented jagged ideological divisions in our nation.

Like a humpback's song, communal laments are highly organized. There are generally six parts:

1. *The address*, which is often something like "Hear Me, O God"
2. *The lament proper*, a brief explanation of why the people need God's assistance
3. *The confession of trust*, when the people affirm that they believe God will hear their prayers

4. *The petition*, which is the "ask" of what the people want God to do
5. *The exclamation of certainty*, in which the people affirm that God hears their prayers
6. *Praise*, an offering of thanks for God's intervention

I wonder if the humpbacks have cause for communal lament.

Maybe some of their songs are prayers to their Creator: low growls expressing their sorrow, screeches requesting God's help on their journeys, and siren-like words of thanks for the provision they find in the ocean depths as they make their way home.

◆

Read a paragraph from Steinbeck's The Log from the Sea of Cortez:

Most of the feeling we call religious, most of the mystical outcrying which is one of the most prized and used and desired reactions of our species, is really the understanding and the attempt to say that man is related to the whole thing, related inextricably to all reality, known and unknowable. This is a simple thing to say, but the profound feeling of it made a Jesus, a St. Augustine, a

St. Francis, a Roger Bacon, a Charles Darwin, and an Einstein. Each of them in his own tempo and with his own voice discovered and reaffirmed with astonishment the knowledge that all things are one thing and that one thing is all things—plankton, a shimmering phosphorescence on the sea and the spinning planets and an expanding universe, all bound together by the elastic string of time. It is advisable to look from the tide pool to the stars and then back to the tide pool again.

◆

Take a moment to sit or lie back, and get completely comfortable. Allow your shoulders to drop, and relax your legs and hips. Let your jaw softly open. Take a full breath into your belly, and exhale with sound.

Tonight, as you prepare to sleep, imagine a humpback whale singing a song of lament on your behalf, deep down below the surface of the ocean.

Imagine him floating.

Listen for this mystical outcrying, echoing for miles for all the creatures under the sea to hear.

Hear him growl and roar.

Listen to him sigh and whine.

What might he be asking on your behalf?

What might he hope for you?

What are your best hopes for him?

Reflect on your own connectedness with all the plants and creatures that live in the ocean, including a humpback singing his own strange and particular song.

Think of him with an open heart.

Imagine the stars, scattered like glitter in the night sky, shining down on you both tonight.

4
MANGROVE FORESTS

THE ROOTS OF LOVE

Perhaps it's the whimsical name J. N. "Ding" Darling National Wildlife Refuge. Or the otherworldly quiet of the place in Sanibel Island, Florida. Maybe it's the fact that the forest grows along the edge of shallow salt water, tree roots and branches teeming with thousands of tiny crabs. Whatever it is, when you kayak through the mangrove forest—having started off at the canoe launch in Tarpon Bay, ever on the lookout for manatees—well, it may leave you feeling like you are on another planet.

Lines from Lewis Carroll's *Jabberwocky* might come to mind. The poem begins (and ends) with this line: "'Twas brillig, and the slithy toves / Did gyre and gimble in the wabe; / All mimsy were the borogoves, / And the mome raths outgrabe." *Mangroves. Tarpon Bay. "Ding" Darling. Manatees.* These sound like they could be figments of Carroll's imagination. *Slithy toves* and *mome raths*? Perhaps they lurk here in the Florida swamps as well.

Paddling through the wildlife refuge does more than evoke Carroll's nonsense rhymes. To navigate around narrow turns and away from low-hanging branches in the watery path requires focus. The fact that there are alligators in these shallow waters adds a sense of uncertain danger, as do those scuttling black crabs that stream down tree branches and scurry through their exposed roots.

As you lift your paddle, you stay silent, watchful for egrets, cormorants, and herons. No phones ring or chime; nothing calls your attention away from the moment and place where you are. Your paddling is almost meditative. You are *present*.

Although John Steinbeck, in *The Log from the Sea of Cortez*, insists that "no one likes" the mangroves, they're magical to me. Maybe the ones in Florida are more beautiful than those he visited, which he said were riddled with insects and mud and disgusting smells.

Mangroves thrive in warm, tropical areas where salt and fresh water come together. Unlike most living things—

and unlike *every other* species of tree—these trees metabolize salt water. They excrete salt through their waxy leaves. One of the few other living things that can tolerate salt water is the albatross, that huge ocean seabird. It drinks salt water; glands behind its eye sockets excrete excess salt in a solution, draining it through the tip of the bird's beak. Sharks and ocean fish process salt water through their kidneys and gills and special glands. But for almost everything that is alive, salt water is toxic.

The root systems of the mangrove trees are tangled and dense, and their three different types of roots serve three purposes. "Breathing roots" are above ground and have pores through which oxygen enters the trees' underground tissues. All plants require oxygen, but there is very little and sometimes no oxygen in the soil in which the mangroves grow. So their breathing roots allow them to receive oxygen from the atmosphere. The second type of mangrove root is the "stilt root." These roots also allow oxygen to enter into the tree, but they serve the additional purpose of propping up the tree by growing deep in the ground, some distance away from the main stem. Mangroves' "vivipary roots" allow the trees to reproduce. (The word *viviparous* means that an organism brings forth live young. Mammals, of course, are viviparous, but how strange that these trees are too.) Seeds are germinated and develop into seedlings while they are still attached to the parent tree, which supplies the seedling with needed water and nutrients. These later detach and float away to find suitable soil to root in. Another plant that is viviparous is the tiger lily, as it also produces seeds that germinate before detaching from the parent plant.

Not only do mangrove roots allow for reproduction and protect them against high winds and storms and the ebb and flow of the tide, but their underwater roots offer protective habitats for just-hatched fish and sharks. Shrimp, crabs, and other species often begin their lives in "mangrove root nurseries," where they are shielded from predators. Mangroves also filter and remove pollutants from water and protect the shoreline against erosion, safeguarding natural habitats as well as human-made housing and infrastructure.

Mangrove forests are worthy warriors in the fight against climate change; they store vast amounts of carbon in their leaves, trunks, and soil. Carbon storage in marine plants is known as "blue carbon" and is a strategy scientists and policy experts believe helps mitigate the atmospheric carbon that leads to global climate change. It's no wonder, then, that mangroves are sometimes nicknamed "coastline defenders" or "bioshields." In Sanibel, Florida, for all of those reasons and more—including the forests' value to tourism—the state's nearly five hundred thousand acres of mangrove swamp are cherished and protected.

Emerging from the kayak trail down Commodore Creek and back out onto Tarpon Bay, you'll probably want to reach for a pair of sunglasses. The light reflecting off the open water is a surprise; the mangroves have been a canopy, shielding you from the brightness of the sun. Stop paddling for a few moments and let the waves direct you. The water will slap up against the kayak. Let your boat float for a while, and enjoy the feeling of the sun's rays warming you and of rocking back and forth gently in the sea.

◆

Read the following words by John Main, a British Roman Catholic priest and monk. Before entering the priesthood, Main was a civil servant who worked in Kuala Lumpur, Malaysia. A Hindu monk there taught him meditation and how to use a mantra to experience "mindful stillness." (A mantra is a short sound, word, or phrase repeated and used in meditation or relaxation practices to help focus the attention.) Main returned to the United Kingdom, was ordained, and began Christian meditation groups using what he learned from his swami friend in Malaysia. In his book The Inner Christ, *Main wrote, "Just as the roots of trees hold the soil firm and stop erosion, so it is with the roots of love that hold the ground of our being together. They provide the context in which we live and grow. And they trace us back to God as the first root of all being."*

◆

Main suggested spending twenty to thirty minutes every morning and night in meditation. When starting a meditation or prayer practice for the first time, setting a timer for three minutes and building up to a longer contemplative time can be a good way to begin.

Main recommended using the word maranatha *as a mantra, slowly saying each of the four syllables. In the biblical tradition,* maranatha *is an Aramaic word that means "Come, O Lord"— although Main said it's not important to think about the meaning of a mantra when you are repeating it. If you don't connect with that word, choose another, such as* mystery, merciful, *or* miracle. *You could also choose to repeat a short sentence.*

Borrowing from Main, you could repeat, "The roots of love hold me" or "I am rooted in love."

Tonight, as you move toward sleep, consider silently repeating a mantra or prayer phrase to center your thoughts and calm your spirit. Sit back or lie down. Get completely comfortable. Take a few deep breaths so you can relax deeply and remain still for a few minutes. Begin your mantra. You can speak it aloud softly or just repeat it in your mind.

If thoughts and images come to mind or distract you, don't worry; simply acknowledge them and then imagine them floating off like a waxy leaf from a mangrove tree out to sea. Return yourself gently to your mantra.

Keep returning to your repeated prayer word or phrase, spoken silently, reciting it in your mind. If you fall asleep when you're repeating your mantra, be grateful for the rest.

Remember, like the roots of the mangrove tree hold, feed, and protect, the roots of love hold you.

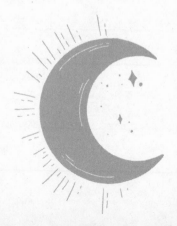

5
HUMMINGBIRDS

A GLITTERING, A SHIMMER, A TUNE

You are likely familiar with many quirky, collective nouns for creatures: a *pod* of dolphins, a *pack* of wolves, a *school* of fish. Those are all orderly enough terms. But what about a *squabble* of seagulls, a *murmuration* of starlings, a *consortium* of crabs, a *kaleidoscope* of butterflies, or a *shrewdness* of apes? The fact that we assign such amiable names to groups of animals, birds, and other creatures may be one sign of biophilia: our deep affinity and love for all that is alive.

Aside from my very favorite—the nearly ludicrous *implausibility* of gnus (gnus!)—some of the best names for a grouping of creatures are given to hummingbirds. You can refer to them collectively as a *bouquet*, a *glittering*, a *hover*, a *shimmer*, a *charm*, or a *tune*. Those words all point to the magic of watching hummingbirds in motion, the way they arrive at a flower or feeder—as though by teleportation—and then disappear in an instant. As the only birds that can fly forward and backward, they can also hover and even fly upside down. They interact with each other seemingly playfully, as though they are in a game of freeze tag or hide-and-seek.

It's no wonder that in many cultures, hummingbirds are considered supernatural. The Mayans believed that the sun went about in disguise as a hummingbird, and one of the two main deities in the Aztec religion was represented as one. Throughout history and across cultures, seeing a hummingbird has been considered a sign of good luck or even that a loved one is visiting from the afterlife.

Hummingbirds get their name from the humming sound their wings make as they beat them up to two hundred times per second. There is an old story—likely fictional—that the sound of lightsabers in *Star Wars* movies (*voommm, vvvvvrrroom*) was based on the whirring sound of hummingbird wings. North American hummingbirds average about fifty-three beats per second in flight, and they reach speeds of up to thirty miles per hour while flying and up to sixty miles per hour when diving.

There are more than three hundred species of hummingbirds globally. They are some of the smallest birds and weigh about as much as a penny; their nests are about the size of a golf ball and their eggs the size of green peas or navy beans. They use fine plant fibers, including dandelion seeds, to build their nests, and they stretch sticky spider silk around them to hold them together. Most hummingbird females lay two eggs, which they incubate for fifteen to eighteen days; the young juveniles leave the nest eighteen to twenty-eight days after hatching.

Fewer than two dozen species of hummingbirds are found in North America, and in Illinois, where I live, the most common is the ruby-throated hummingbird. The male of this species has, as his name describes, a striking red throat. He also sports a white collar and has a shiny green back. Females also have green backs and white, black, and grayish-green tail feathers. When they arrive in my part of the country, we know that spring is on the way.

One night this past summer while we were making dinner, my husband, David, and I chatted about hummingbirds. That day, I'd seen at least a dozen arrive at and then disappear from my friend's backyard feeder as we lingered over lunch.

"It was hard to concentrate on our conversation," I told David. "They were just so—what's even the word—*exquisite? Magical? Iridescent?*"

David had nodded and mm-hmmed.

Later that night, he looked up from reading the news on his phone and said with conviction, "You know what it is?"

"What *what* is?" I asked.

"Hummingbirds," he said, as though no time had passed since we were talking about them. "So we know birds descended from dinosaurs. But think about it: I mean, the difference between hummingbirds—those colors and the way they flit and fly—and a big T. rex stomping around? Well, it's a miracle."

He corrected himself: "No, it's a whimsical *delight* of a miracle."

Then he fell silent again and went back to reading.

Whimsical, delightful, a miracle: yes, all of the above.

Hummingbirds visit more than two thousand flowers per day. Despite their size, they're intelligent; their brains compose proportionally more of their body weight than any other bird's. (Their brains make up more than 4 percent of their body weight; human brains make up about 2 percent of ours.) Studies indicate that hummingbirds can remember *every single flower* they've ever drunk from. They can even recognize human faces, sometimes flying close to the people who feed them, swooping in to alert their human caretakers when feeders are empty.

Loners in the world of birds, hummingbirds don't migrate in flocks (so, sadly, we don't often have occasion to use those playful terms for groups of them). They typically travel on their own for hundreds of miles.

Hummingbirds can not only see every color that we can, but they can process ultraviolet light, thus seeing colors we cannot. Human eyes are "trichromatic," meaning we have three types of cones, while many other creatures have four. Hummingbirds see ultraviolet wavelength. In other words, they see colors we can't even begin to *imagine*!

You may have been taught, like I was, that hummingbirds use their tongues like straws to suck up nectar. The way they drink, however, is more intricate than that. They have forked tongues lined with ultrafine extensions called lamellae. When a hummingbird starts to drink, its tongue extends into the flower, the fork opens, and the lamellae unfurl to capture the nectar. The bird then brings its tongue back into its mouth to ingest the nectar. Hummingbirds' metabolisms, given the speed at which they fly, are incredibly efficient. To keep their bodies fueled, they eat about every ten minutes. And they consume up to two to three times their body weight in nectar and bugs every single day.

Hummingbirds also seem to enjoy playing. Although researchers explain that some of what might *look* like play to humans is territorial behavior, there seems to be an undeniable element of flirtatious fun—as is true with many other birds—in their courting. Males engage in mating dances, puffing out their chests to show off their colors. Male hummingbirds' two common courtship displays are called the "dive display" and the "shuttle display." In a dive display, a male tries to capture a female bird's attention by climbing 60–130 feet into the air and then nosediving down while making what has been described as a "honking" sound. A shuttle display is more nuanced and, you might say, quietly seductive. In it, a male hummingbird will fly back and forth before a female, swinging his body and singing a gentler song. Whether she has been presented with a dive or shuttle display, the female will indicate her interest in a particular male by alighting and landing on a nearby branch and spreading her tail feathers.

Smart, distinctive, elegant, and even sensual: choosing only one way to describe this group of amazing birds doesn't seem important. Hummingbirds are all at once a bouquet, a glittering, a hover, a shimmer, a charm, *and* a tune.

◆

Genevieve Taggard was an American poet born at the very end of the nineteenth century who wrote more than a dozen volumes of poetry, a biography of Emily Dickinson, and several other books. She was an activist for social justice who spoke out power-fully against inequality, especially what was experienced by people most affected by the Great Depression. Her first book of poetry, For Eager Lovers, *was published in 1922.*

Read the poem "Questions" by Taggard:

Never heard happier laughter.
Where did you hear it?
Somewhere in the future.
Very far in the future?
No, not far, but near. American
Laughter. Listen,

From this laughter tumbling in a river
We will make our peace (true peace)
our wealth (true wealth)
And our justice (true justice).

◆

Tonight, as you put the day's activity behind you and get ready to sleep, reflect on Taggard's poem. She indicates that true peace, true wealth, and true justice are somehow born of laughter. How does that strike you? Perhaps it sounds as unlikely and mysterious and delightful as a hummingbird descending from a dinosaur.

Tonight, take a few deep, steady breaths.

Before you go off to sleep, practice a short smiling meditation. Yes, that's a real thing! Just smiling, even if you're not "feeling it," reduces stress hormones and activates hormones that accelerate healing, reduce pain, and improve your mood.

A smiling meditation is as simple as it sounds.

Take a deep breath in through your nose and out through your mouth.

Relax the muscles in your face, and smile.

Imagine laughter flowing like a river or hovering above you like a hummingbird over a flower.

6
ST. PAUL'S ROCKS

A WILDLY WONDERFUL WORLD

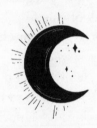

A couple of years ago, *National Geographic* magazine included photographs of a newly discovered fish in the Atlantic Ocean off the coast of Brazil. Named *Aphrodite anthias*, this little creature looks as if a preschooler wielding a fistful of neon highlighters joyfully dotted and striped a common goldfish in purple, yellow, pink, and green. One reporter quipped that it had a "ridiculous 80's-themed color palette." Maybe I'm alone here, but I was truly surprised when I read this story: We're *still* discovering new species of fish? Also, I thought, What is "ridiculous" about a palette from the 1980s?

The researchers who discovered this fish found nothing silly about it. In fact, they sound quite reverent when they discuss it. One said, "While we were collecting the Aphrodite anthias, a large Six-gill shark (*Hexanchus griseus*) came very close to both of us, but that didn't divert our attention from the new, exquisitely beautiful species, and we never even saw the shark. The beauty of the Aphrodite anthias enchanted us during its discovery much like Aphrodite's beauty enchanted ancient Greek gods."

Looking at pictures of this fish, I remember my husband's standard response after our children ate popsicles from the ice cream truck when they were little. Catching sight of their mouths stained neon pink or blue, he'd say, "Whoa, there! Now those are colors we do *not* find in nature." I'd laugh and agree. Looking at photographs of this wackily colored fish, I see that we were wrong.

Aphrodite anthias was discovered in 2017, at a depth of nearly four hundred feet, at what's known as the St. Peter and St. Paul Archipelago—or, more commonly, "St. Paul's Rocks." This tiny bundle of islands, about seven hundred miles northeast of Brazil, comprises six larger islands, four smaller ones, and several rock tops. St. Paul's Rocks was discovered in 1511 by a Brazilian ship called the *São Pedro* (thus the "St. Peter" in the archipelago's longer name), which had lost its way and crashed into them. It was out in the middle of nowhere; the ship would have had no reason to expect to collide with *anything* there. The crew of the *São Pedro* would eventually be rescued by a ship called the *São Pablo* (or the "St. Paul," thus completing the name of the place).

This little knot of rocks has had some famous visitors, including Charles Darwin. In 1831, a young Darwin began his five-year voyage around the world in HMS *Beagle*, collecting and studying animal, plant, and rock samples. Over the course of his journey, he observed that different parts of the world contain *similar* animals and plants, but he noted differences too and began to surmise that living things adapt in order to best thrive and survive in their local environments. Darwin continued to develop these ideas; they underpin his theories of evolution and natural selection.

Darwin and the *Beagle* stopped at St. Paul's Rocks on February 16, 1832. He recorded his thoughts in his journal, calling it a "cluster of rocks" that "rises abruptly out of the depths of the ocean." Modern-day geologists marvel that Darwin, on his brief visit there, correctly noted that unlike almost all other islands on the open ocean, St. Paul's Rocks is not composed of coral or lava. (Hawaii, for example, is the product of millions of years of volcanic eruptions deep underwater that built and built until the islands finally reached the ocean's surface.) Instead, Darwin determined that St. Paul's Rocks, rising more than four thousand meters up from the ocean floor, is the product of geologic uplift. The rocks are not coral or volcanic material but silicates: part of the earth's mantle that has been pushed up by shifting tectonic plates.

On these islands, Darwin found a few insects, little vegetation, and two types of birds, both of which still live there. He wrote, "We found on St. Paul's only two kinds of birds—the booby and the noddy. . . . Both are of a tame and stupid disposition." The archipelago is forbidding. Only one of the islets, called Belmonte, has any vegetation to speak of. The others are mostly barren and only home to the seabirds Darwin observed, some crabs, and insects.

St. Paul's Rocks is uninhabited by humans except for the researchers who work at the science station established there in 1998. It's a rich area for marine biologists, in large part because its reefs boast some of the highest levels of endemism in the Atlantic. When something is endemic to a certain place, it cannot be found anywhere else in the world. Seven fish—including the oblique butterfly fish and the salmon-spotted jewelfish—are exclusively found there. On its discovery, Aphrodite anthias became the eighth fish known to be endemic to St. Paul's Rocks.

So why are reef fish so colorful and rich with distinct patterns? After all, the "tame and stupid" boobies and noddies to which Darwin so comically referred are more unfussy in their uniform of black, white, and brown—just the same colors of the rocks on which they nest and live. Given the bright colors and plants of a coral reef, is it that their colors and patterns also serve as effective camouflage, protecting the fish from predators? Does it have to do with the way light is filtered underwater? Is it because they live so far under the surface of the ocean, where more colors are absorbed? Are their palettes so "ridiculous" and "80's-themed" because reef fish see differently than we do? Does it help them attract mates?

I can't pretend to know, and researchers continue to probe this question, but I can celebrate their wild colors and their whimsical names. And I expect that before long, marine biologists at St. Paul's Rocks will find another new species, one not found anywhere else in the world.

That makes me feel hopeful, expectant even, knowing there are more beautiful, dazzling mysteries yet to be discovered.

♦

Read Psalm 104:24–26 (MSG):

What a wildly wonderful world, God!
You made it all, with Wisdom at your side,
made earth overflow with your wonderful creations.
Oh, look—the deep, wide sea,
brimming with fish past counting,
sardines and sharks and salmon.
Ships plow those waters,
and Leviathan, your pet dragon, romps in them.

◆

The two researchers who discovered Aphrodite anthias at St. Paul's Rocks were so taken with it that they didn't even notice a huge shark swimming just over their heads.

Tonight, as you relax and prepare for sleep, consider this:

When has something struck you as so beautiful or so colorful that you lost sight of yourself or where you were?

What colors in nature dazzle you? Leaves on a tree in autumn, in their red and orange and yellow? Tropical fish in a tank? A sunrise, or a sunset? The crystalline blue of the ocean? A lilac bush in spring? A butterfly's wings?

Allow your imagination to flit from image to image from the list above and perhaps others that enter your mind.

As you drift off, imagine the still-undiscovered species of fish around St. Paul's Rocks, off the coast of Brazil, way out on its own in the Atlantic Ocean.

Know that there are undiscovered parts of you too: dazzling mysteries deep below the surface.

There are colors and patterns and qualities in you that will emerge, like exquisite little fish suddenly appearing to a diver. Let them take you by surprise.

7
HONEY

A BEEHIVE HERE INSIDE MY HEART

My daughter and I weave through the aisles of the farmers' market, sidestepping strollers, pausing to greet neighbors and friends, and bending to give dogs a pat. We occasionally get separated and lose sight of each other for a moment in the swarm of people, but then we spot each other again.

In one stall, a nun wearing a traditional habit and a silver crucifix sells the baguettes, fruit tarts, and croissants that she and her sisters have made at their convent nearby. She's French, her accent thick as she tells us she's happy to see us again. She slips two chocolate croissants into a white paper bag and neatly folds the top, almost singing the words "Merci!" and "God bless you" as we move on.

Squeezing past a cluster of people waiting to buy sweet corn, I notice another farm's offering of pints of blackberries and mounds of eggplants, beets, and red cabbage. It is a study in purple. I think of the Impressionists, who were so obsessed with the color that art critics in their day accused them of suffering from "violettomania." The painter Claude Monet was undeterred—which won't surprise anyone who knows his work. "I have finally discovered the true color of the atmosphere," he said. "It's violet. Fresh air is violet."

Then we reach the beekeeper. Jars of amber honey glow in the sunlight on the table in front of him—they're electric. The beekeeper's subtle smile almost makes it seem like he's resisting the urge to brag. My daughter chooses a honey straw, raspberry flavored, and I buy honey crystals to stir into my tea. The beekeeper hands me the jar of crystals, cradling it with both of his hands. For a moment, I think he's going to rescind the sale, like a painter who's so in love with his work that he refuses to part with it.

I can't blame him. Honey *is* precious, and it's good for the heart. Some studies report that honey is a better treatment for nighttime coughing than the kind of suppressants most of us pick up at the drugstore. Archaeologists who have found pots of it while excavating ancient Egyptian tombs say its shelf life is "eternal." It never goes bad, even after a container has been opened.

Describing the strange way honey is made requires citing a rapid-fire succession of very large and very small numbers. To make a pound of honey, for example, bees must gather nectar from two million flowers. One bee, in its brief lifetime of only a few weeks, only makes about a twelfth of a teaspoon. And although a honeybee's brain is about the size of a sesame seed, its ability to learn, remember, and communicate is astonishing. When bees return from collecting nectar to their colonies—consisting of about twenty thousand to sixty thousand bees—they engage in what beekeepers call a "waggle dance," which tells the others the exact distance and direction of flowers that will yield still more pollen and nectar. This dance also reveals where water can be found.

In Scripture, honey is repeatedly a symbol of God's goodness. The promised land flowed "with milk and honey" (Exodus 3:8), although some scholars now say it was probably date or fig nectar, not honey from bees, that "flowed" there. John the Baptist survived on honeycomb. And Proverbs 16:24 compares "pleasant words" to a honeycomb: "sweet to the soul, and health to the bones" (KJV). Elsewhere in Proverbs, we're told to eat honey, for it is good and "sweet to the taste" (Proverbs 24:13 NLT).

The goodness of honey goes beyond taste. It has been used as a beauty product for thousands of years; Cleopatra's beauty regimen is said to have included applying honey to her face and bathing in milk and honey. Over the centuries, honey has been used to treat wounds because of its antiseptic properties. Honey can provide a quick burst of energy, and researchers now also claim that it reduces stress levels and can even prevent memory loss.

Eating a spoonful of honey before bed is a centuries' old practice in many cultures around the world. It prevents plaque from forming on teeth, boosts the immune system, helps prevent acid reflux, stabilizes blood sugar levels, and contributes to the release of melatonin, which is known as the "sleep hormone." Melatonin promotes healthy sleep, orients our sleep-wake cycles, and helps recover and rebuild body tissues during sleep. Try a spoonful of honey sometime just before you go to bed.

Amina Harris, executive director of the Honey and Pollination Center at the University of California, calls bees "magical." On their forays into the fields, worker bees collect nectar in special sacks in their stomachs. Back at the hive, they then remove the nectar by passing it by mouth to other bees, who then chew on it for about half an hour. Harris explains that part of why honey never spoils has to do with an enzyme in bees' stomachs. When the bees pass the nectar to each other by mouth, the enzyme mixes with it, changing its properties and giving it that "eternal" shelf life.

The processed nectar is then moved into the honeycomb, but the job's not yet done. Nectar is 60 to 80 percent water and honey only about 14 to 18 percent, so the bees must dry out the nectar. They do so by flapping their wings—at twelve thousand beats per minute. This creates their signature buzzing sound and, more importantly, turns the nectar into sticky honey. The bees then store the honey in the cells of the hive and seal each cell with a thin layer of beeswax.

But what's the story with those perfect six-sided cells that hold the queen bee's eggs and store the honey? How and why do bees create the honeycombs the way they do? Researchers don't agree on what is the exact process. We know the cells begin as circles, but then, some scientists say, the bees use heat from their bodies to melt the wax into perfect hexagons. But what scientists *do* know is that a grid of hexagons is the most resourceful use of materials. In the construction of their honeycombs, bees create the most durable structure and the largest possible number of storage units—and use the least amount of wax.

Bees work hard. They communicate with each other by dancing. They build stunning, efficient honeycombs. And they keep us alive by pollinating the plants that will reproduce and grow and be harvested and fill the shelves of grocery stores or sit in gorgeous heaps under the canopies at farmers' markets.

No wonder the beekeeper is so proud.

Home from our outing, I open the jar of honey crystals and spoon a tiny amount on the tip of my tongue. I let them dissolve, and the sweetness fills my mouth.

◆

Read these lines from the poem "Last Night as I Was Sleeping"
by Antonio Machado. You might not be familiar with Machado's
work, but you've likely come across some version of his sentiment:
"There is no path, the path is made by walking," taken from his
poem known in English as "Wayfarer, the Only Way" or "Traveler,
Your Footprints" and paraphrased from the Spanish in many
different forms. Machado was one of the most important literary
figures in Spain in the twentieth century. Reflective and spiritual,
Machado's poetry focuses on dreams and on the natural beauty
of his homeland.

Last Night as I Was Sleeping

Last night as I was sleeping,
I dreamt—marvelous error!—
that a spring was breaking
out in my heart.
I said: Along which secret aqueduct,
Oh water, are you coming to me,
water of a new life
that I have never drunk?

Last night as I was sleeping,
I dreamt—marvelous error!—
that I had a beehive

here inside my heart.
And the golden bees
were making white combs
and sweet honey
from my old failures.

Last night as I was sleeping,
I dreamt—marvelous error!—
that a fiery sun was giving
light inside my heart.
It was fiery because I felt
warmth as from a hearth,
and sun because it gave light
and brought tears to my eyes.

Last night as I slept,
I dreamt—marvelous error!—
that it was God I had
here inside my heart.

◆

The poet dreams he has a spring, a beehive, a fiery sun, and God inside his heart.

Let your body relax, taking a deep breath in and exhaling even longer. Imagine what it would feel like to have each of these things in your heart.

What would a spring *feel like?*
A beehive?
A sun?
God?

The poet dreams that "golden bees" are making honey from his failures. Imagine something good and sweet being made from the broken pieces of your own life. Picture something good happening inside your heart while you are sleeping tonight. Something will be healed. Something new will be created, and it will be something sweet.

There is nothing you need to do to make this happen. Just rest, and let the golden bees do their good work inside of you.

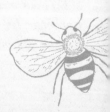

8
THE OVERVIEW EFFECT

THE BACKDROP OF THE UNIVERSE

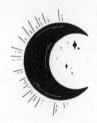

In an interview for *Sick in the Head: Conversations about Life and Comedy*, a book by director and screenwriter Judd Apatow, Jerry Seinfeld discloses two surprising facts about himself. Not only has he maintained a faithful meditation practice for many years ("*Serenity now!*"), but he hung photographs taken by the Hubble telescope on the walls of the writers' room while working on *Seinfeld*. He said he did this so he'd keep perspective; the photos from outer space were there to remind him how insignificant he was. Seinfeld says these images would calm him down when he started taking himself too seriously, thinking that what he was doing was "important." In the book, Apatow responds that this would make him feel depressed, but Seinfeld says experiencing a sense of insignificance feels uplifting to him.

I relate to this: insignificance feels *freeing* to me. It is like a hall pass, a permission slip, a get-out-of-jail-free card in the game of Monopoly. Remembering how small I am—letting go of the misguided belief that my decisions, my right thinking, and the details of my life are all critical—is a gift. It allows me to hit the reset button and get at least a bit closer to being on track, mentally and spiritually.

I think of the psalmist who writes,

> *When I look at your heavens,*
> *the work of your fingers,*
> *the moon and the stars that you have established;*
> *what are human beings that you are mindful of them,*
> *mortals that you care for them?*
>
> —Psalm 8:3–4

I don't feel belittled or depressed when reading those words but honored. Relieved. I let a deep breath out. I'm reminded that I'm very small, and the Divine is hundreds of universes and galaxies more significant than me. *Mysterious. Massive. Other.*

Of course, while looking at photographs of outer space captured by a telescope is moving, how much more awe inspiring would it actually be to see it in person? I can't imagine it! But I love to read accounts of what has been called "the overview effect": that cognitive shift people experience when they have viewed the earth from space. They describe the feeling of seeing our planet from that perspective as a kind of ecstasy. Space tourists and astronauts report that the overview effect makes the things that they worried about before that moment disappear, and they report having a new or renewed desire to protect the earth and to be in peaceful communion with all of its people.

One astrophysicist writes, "When in space, astronauts have repeatedly reported inexplicable euphoria, a 'cosmic connection' or an increased sensitivity to their place in the Universe. The experience sounds like the ultimate high, or the ultimate enlightening; it would appear that without try-ing, astronauts are able to attain a similar mental state as meditating Buddhist monks." (Remember John Steinbeck's marine biologist friend Ed Ricketts, who saw *everything* as interrelated? He, too, achieved this kind of enlightenment despite being confined to planet earth, exploring only the universe of the ocean.)

Self-proclaimed "space philosopher" and author Frank White invented the term *the overview effect* in 1987. White's interest in outer space began, he has said, when he was ten years old and someone gave him a book titled *Stars*. He later graduated from Harvard University, attended Oxford University on a Rhodes scholarship, and wrote several books about space exploration. He has received many accolades from the scientific community, but you wouldn't know all of this from doing a quick internet search on his name. His online presence, fittingly, is small and quite understated. "I am interested in space exploration and human evolution," his Twitter handle reads. It seems he has a comfortable relationship with where he stands in the universe; he's not trying to prove or assert his significance.

Common features of having experienced the overview effect include feelings of awe, an understanding of the interconnectedness of all living things, and a sense of responsibility for the environment. White was inspired with this idea while on a cross-country plane trip as a young man. Looking out the windows on the land below, he wondered what it would be like to have an overview of the entire earth from outer space. Later, he'd talk with astronauts about what it was like for them actually to experience it.

On a blog, White discussed how various astronauts described the overview effect:

> The first thing that most people think about when they think about the overview effect is no borders or boundaries on the Earth. And we know that. . . . But it's knowing intellectually versus experiencing it. There's also the striking thinness of the

atmosphere, something that they see. And again, for most astronauts, the feeling that the Earth itself is a whole system, and we're just a part of it. We need to think of ourselves as part of this organic system, if you will. . . . We are really all in this together. Our fate is bound up with people that we may think are really different. . . . We may have different religions, we may have different politics. But ultimately, we are connected. Totally connected. And not only with people, but with life. We're totally connected with life. And everything relates to everything else.

White has also said that it's difficult to describe the experience because words fall short when a person tries to describe seeing the earth "against the backdrop of the universe."

You and I might consider, Would seeing the earth hanging in that backdrop of space make us reconsider the notion of boundaries and borders? How might we differently perceive our divisions and our wars? How might we redefine who's "in" and who's "out" in terms of our families and communities? How might binary definitions of so many kinds fail to make sense or be meaningful anymore?

How might we choose to live and move on this planet in new ways were we to witness its true vulnerability—that thin line of atmosphere that shields us from the sun's harsh rays?

How might we embrace calm and gain new perspective on both the importance and the insignificance of our individual lives?

How might our hearts lift, in praise, to the Divine?

◆

Teresa of Ávila was a Spanish contemplative in the fifteenth century. Witty, smart, and born into an affluent family, she was taught to read and write, unlike many women of her time. In her writing, she admits to being a flirt—but she never married, refusing to enter into an arranged marriage as a young woman. Instead, she entered religious life. Over the course of her life as a nun, her faith waxed and waned, but when she was forty, she had a profound religious experience and many visions of God. Devout and outspoken after these experiences, she kept her sense of humor, boldly expressing her impatience with self-righteous members of the church. One of her most famous quotes, which may actually be fictitious, is, "God save us from sour-faced saints!" Her books are classics in Christian mysticism and are full of wisdom and assurance.

Read these lines by St. Teresa of Ávila:

Nothing move thee;
Nothing terrify thee;
Everything passes;
God never changes.
Patience be to thee.

◆

Sit in silence for a few minutes, just breathing gently.

Now imagine seeing the earth from far above; envision that famous "blue marble" picture of our planet, a perfect circle, the black backdrop of outer space behind and around it. Imagine that inky depth of space in which it hangs. See the swirl of white clouds, the patches of blues and greens and browns spread over the earth's face.

Next, imagine where you are located in that picture. Know, with quiet confidence, that you are one tiny life, occupying one tiny place. While your life is precious, you are blessedly insignificant.

Remember, as St. Teresa reminds us, that everything passes. Now isn't forever. This moment isn't every moment. This place isn't every place.

God and this universe are much, much bigger than we are.

Breathe out any worries and fears; breathe in a sense of calm. Repeat silently, in your mind, phrases that bring you peace. They could be the following:

May I be content.

May I be safe.

May I feel God's presence.

May I remember that everything passes.

May I rest well tonight.

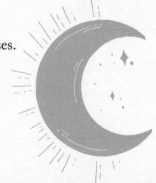

9

MONTSERRAT MOUNTAIN

MY SENSES QUICKEN AND GROW DEEP

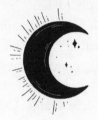

Considered a sacred place for centuries, with rocky spires that reach toward the sky, Montserrat mountain has a captivating history. Some forty-five million years ago, the area just outside of Barcelona, Spain, was mostly covered by an inland sea that flowed to the Mediterranean. The rivers that fed into those waters deposited rock, limestone, and other material there. When the earth's plates shifted twenty-five million years ago, the rocks and limestone were driven upward and the water out to sea, creating the mountain. Over the next millions of years, exposed to the wind and weather, the mountain was molded and shaped by erosion, and Montserrat was fashioned into the strange sight we see today.

Montserrat is of great interest to geologists, and when they describe it, they often talk about its unconformities. These are gaps in the geologic record; when two layers of rock come together but they are found to be from much different time periods, it's dubbed an "unconformity." Unconformities can be caused by erosion, shifting tectonic plates, or other factors. Sometimes the place where these two disparate layers of rock come together is tilted. Sometimes two very different types of rocks—sedimentary with, say, igneous rock—from different periods are enigmatically layered together, or there's other evidence of disruption. Some of Montserrat's peaks look sharp and jagged, like a knife. Others almost look like human forms and bring to mind the mo'ai, those blunt carved statues on Easter Island, with their thick heads and wide torsos. Still other areas of the mountain look gently rounded as though they've been shaped with wet sand and left to dry. While Montserrat itself might remember its past, earth scientists know there is much more to its story than the geologic record shows.

Called Mons Serratus (Saw-Toothed Mountain) by the Romans and Montsagrat (Sacred Mountain) by the Catalans, the unusual rock formations have also been given a more mystical explanation, one that endures to this day. A medieval legend claims that the mountain was formed when angels came down from heaven bearing a golden saw to carve a throne for the Virgin Mary. The mountain's peculiar beauty—as well as its history, rich with supernatural sightings and episodes—makes this seem, well, plausible.

The mountain has a long memory. Even before the time of Christ, Montserrat was a holy site; the Romans built a temple there to worship Venus, the goddess of love. Caves in the mountain were inhabited since prehistoric times. Researchers have long known, given the evidence found there—including bones and broken pottery—that the caves were occupied in Neolithic times. More recently, older artifacts like tools made of flint were discovered that prove that hunter-gatherers also took shelter in those caves twelve to fifteen thousand years ago.

The Holy Grotto, one of the hundred caves of Montserrat, has a long history of sightings of Mary. A text written in the thirteenth century states that on a Saturday evening in the year 880 CE, a group of shepherd children saw a "great light" fall on the mountain and then heard a woman singing. It was the Virgin Mary. The children returned the following week with their parents, and the same events occurred. Clerics, bishops, and others, hearing of this, also visited and witnessed the light and heard the song.

About that time, a wooden statue of the Virgin Mary was found in a cave there. This statue was thought to have been carved in Jerusalem by early Christians. Some even say it was St. Luke who carved her. The bishop of Barcelona had been given it on a journey to Jerusalem, and he brought it home with him. When Spain was invaded in the seventh century, however, the statue was removed from Barcelona and hidden in the mountain for safekeeping. It would remain there for two hundred years, only to be discovered when those shepherd children saw the light shine on the mountain at dusk and heard the Virgin's song. The discovery of the statue and the visitation witnessed by so many made Montserrat into a significant religious destination. St. Ignatius of Loyola made an annual pilgrimage to Montserrat, and typically, more than a million visitors come to the abbey every year, many to ask for the Virgin Mary to heal them or grant them some other blessing.

Founded and built in the eleventh century, the Santa María de Montserrat abbey is now home to more than seventy monks. The church and chapels contain many exquisite sculptures, paintings, mosaics, and other religious artifacts. The abbey is most famous for its twelfth-century Black Madonna, a replica of the original statue from Jerusalem that had been found in the mountain. The Black Madonna sits high above the altar, holding the Christ child and extending her arm. In her hand, she holds a sphere that represents the universe. She is carved in wood, and over time, she has become black, having sat in the presence of burning candles for hundreds of years. She is said to have mystical healing powers and sits behind a sheet of glass, but the hand that holds the universe is exposed; people touch it, asking for her favor.

On a trip to visit one of our children on a college study abroad program, my husband, David, and I take the train to Montserrat. On the hour-long ride, my jet-lagged mind begins to clear as I become present to the unusual beauty of the mountains outside the window. "Now wait," I say to David, keeping my voice low: "What is this place again?" Suddenly, I can't remember if it's a religious site or just a mountain. Why did our son say we needed to visit? Had he said it was a chapel? A forest preserve? A prehistoric site? I would learn that it is, of course, all of these things.

We walk silently around the abbey, peering into the chapels along its sides and stopping to admire paintings and other works of art, but I find myself rushing, eager to be out in those mountains again. They draw me out to them, past the line of pilgrims waiting to climb the steps, to walk above the altar, and to ask for Mary's help. The faces of those in line are weary and tearstained, and I feel the weight of the suffering they carry.

To me, the mountain itself seems a source of healing and consolation, a quiet witness to the passage of time, to the impermanence of our troubles, to the endless creativity and variety of earth's processes. David and I walk the trails above the abbey, the paths bordered by wildflowers, oak trees, and those eccentric rock formations. Geckos scatter as we turn corners and disturb sandy-colored rocks beneath our feet. We silently take in the Mediterranean sky, the hills, and a view of the abbey, like a dollhouse, down below.

Whether it was erosion, chemistry, or even a golden, heavenly saw that carved the peaks of Montserrat, maybe the sound of Mary's voice, singing to those shepherd children, put the finishing touches on the sculpture that is this strange and beautiful mountain.

◆

The Austrian poet Rainer Maria Rilke is one of the most widely read poets today. Loved for his many collections of poetry, Rilke also published a novel and correspondence. His Letters to a Young Poet *is composed of ten letters, written over several years, that he wrote to a nineteen-year-old officer cadet at the same military academy Rilke had attended as a young man. They are full of generous and quotable words of advice about creativity and uncertainty. Take, for instance, "Be patient with all that is unsolved in your heart," "Live the questions," and "Live everything." These letters were written early in his career, not long after Rilke began gaining respect as a poet. His first great work,* The Book of Hours, *was published in 1905, and its theme is the Christian search for God. (The title of the collection refers to illustrated devotional books that contained prayers to be spoken at different times of the day.)*

Read these lines from The Book of Hours*:*

I love my life's dark hours
In which my senses quicken and grow deep,

While, as from faint incense of faded flowers
Or letters old, I magically steep
Myself in days gone by: again I give
Myself unto the past:—again I live.

Now look again at those lines, but just read the last word of each one. Hours. Deep. Flowers. Steep. Give. Live. *Does any one of those words, in particular, speak to you?*

◆

Tonight, in the dark hours as you prepare for sleep, give thought to how, as Rilke puts it, your "senses quicken and grow deep" when you remember the past.

What memories come alive in your imagination when you think about them?

Think back on one positive experience you've had in the past few days. It can be small, like a good cup of coffee. Or it could be more significant, like words of praise from someone you respect or good news about your life or about the state of the world.

Spend some time there, steeping yourself in that good memory.

Involve all your senses, calling to mind the sounds, scents, and sights that surrounded you in that moment, that happy memory.

Say a word of thanks for the gift that is your past, your present, and your future.

10

GINKGOS

THE END OF A LONG DREAM

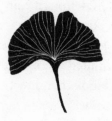

There are more than four thousand species of plants at the arboretum where I'm a member. When I visit, there is one I never miss: the ginkgo. There are more than seventy ginkgo trees there, but I have a favorite, tucked along the side of a path through a grouping of cedars and firs.

Scanning through the photos on my phone, I find dozens of pictures taken from below the branches of this particular tree, pictures taken over the course of several years. It's as though every time I see it, I think that a new set of pictures will somehow be different from the ones I took last month, or last season, or a couple of years ago. Maybe I'm looking for a clue, hoping to gain insight into this tree's personality or to see into its soul. But all my pictures of this tree look almost identical. One branch reaches up and across a swath of blue sky like a banner. The ginkgo's elegant leaves are tiny fans and jade green, except in the autumn, when they are as yellow as a ripe lemon.

I'm sending today's pictures to my friend Jenny, who lives two thousand miles away from me, in Los Angeles. I'm on my own here at the arboretum today and also one of the only people in sight. Things are different here right now, during the pandemic, with limited access to the property and new signage everywhere I look that directs people to keep their distance from one another.

I sit on a low wall to text Jenny. Like my own family, Jenny's has been mostly isolating together for the last year. Her kids are taking their classes online. She and her husband work from home, piecing together their days and weeks, watching the seasons change, and wondering what life will be like after this so-called unprecedented time.

"My favorite ginkgo at the arboretum," I write, sending her a picture. "Checking in on it."

"Gorgeous."

"How's everybody doing?"

"OK. Better."

"Can't believe we were together in January."

"Seems like nine years ago, not months."

"Seriously."

"What in the world did we talk about? What did we even *talk* about before all this?"

"No idea!!!"

I stand up and start walking down the path. Then, as I get deeper into the arboretum, I lose my signal and slip my phone into my jacket pocket.

I turn to look back at my favorite tree. The next time I see it, I imagine it will have turned yellow and dropped its leaves. Of the many things that make ginkgos unique, one is that—unlike other trees—they complete what's called a "synchronized leaf drop" in autumn. The first hard frost of the season causes all of its leaves to fall at once, creating a thick carpet of color on the ground below.

There are hundreds of species of other trees—more than four hundred in the genus *Quercus*, for example, which we know as oaks—but the only species in the genus *Ginkgo* is . . . the *Ginkgo biloba*. So while red oaks (*Quercus rubra*), English oaks (*Quercus robur*), bur oaks (*Quercus macrocarpa*), and all the other oaks produce acorns, have scaly looking bark, and have leaves with deep lobes, the *Ginkgo biloba* is singular, the only child of its genus. When dinosaurs walked the earth, there were several species of *Ginkgo*; now we only have one.

This is why the ginkgo is called a "living fossil," meaning it's the single surviving species of what we know to have been a large group. Its earliest leaf fossils date from 270 million years ago, and there's evidence that at least six other types of ginkgos once existed. Living fossils show little change to their appearance, structure, and function since ancient times. Other examples are horseshoe crabs, platypuses, red pandas, koalas, sandhill cranes, and some tropical palms. All living things adapt to their environments to some extent, of course, so the ginkgo and other "living fossils" are not *identical* to their ancestors, but they are very, very similar.

There are different "cultivars," or bred varieties, of ginkgos, including the Autumn Gold, cultivated for its stunning fall color, and the Princeton Sentry, with a tree shape that is straight and neat and tapers to a tidy point at its top—my favorite tree at the arboretum is one of these. But the *Ginkgo biloba* species has been the same for two hundred million years . . . since before the dinosaurs.

Like many trees, ginkgos are dioecious, meaning that each individual tree is either male or female. Honey locusts, willows, and poplars are dioecious trees too. Other trees, including oaks and pines, are monoecious, meaning one plant can possess both male and female flowers. Ginkgos reproduce when sperm from a male tree connects (via helpful pollinating butterflies and bees) with seeds on a female tree. Interestingly, some ginkgos have been shown to switch sex, from male to female; researchers believe that is a ginkgo's way of ensuring that it will live on.

These trees are survivors. They resist damage from weather, insects, and fungi. They defend themselves by releasing toxins—known in the world of botany as "allelochemicals"—through their leaves when under attack from insects. And in a two-pronged strategy for survival, they can concurrently emit chemicals that attract the infringing insects' predators. They're tolerant of direct sun, drought conditions, and acidity in the soil. After an atomic bomb leveled Hiroshima in 1945, the only living things to survive near the hypocenter were ginkgo trees. Those particular trees are, actually, *still* alive in Japan.

Ginkgos thrive in small spaces and in urban landscapes, adding shade and their refined beauty to cities. The first ginkgo tree in the United States was planted in Philadelphia in 1784 and lived until the 1980s; now you can find them all over the country. Ginkgos can live for thousands of years—some trees in China are more than 2,500 years old. Leaf fossils are abundant in China, and ginkgos were thought to have been extinct until their rediscovery in the late seventeenth century. Happily, they live on.

My loop around the arboretum comes to an end, and I exit into the parking lot. I get into my car, pull off my mask, and look down at my phone. Jenny has texted again, and it's a long one.

"Was just thinking. You know how old people tell stories about how they made it through hard times? Like the Great

Depression or the Dust Bowl or . . . ? Or how we talk about how it was after 9/11? *This* is one of those times. On the other side of this, we'll have gotten through something. We'll always talk about how we managed to make it through."

"It will be good to be on the other side," I reply, letting out a deep, soul-clearing sigh.

I sit in the car and wonder, for a moment, what our changed world will be like. Skimming through the new pictures of my favorite tree, I realize that—in whatever ways society, culture, and even my own life will be changed after this time—one thing will not: the ginkgo tree. Then I rub down my hands with sanitizer, drop my phone into my bag, and begin my drive home.

◆

Matsuo Bashō, a master of haiku in the seventeenth century, is considered one of Japan's greatest poets. A haiku *is a poem comprising three unrhymed lines of five, seven, and five syllables that often includes a seasonal reference and a flash of insight. (In translation, there can be more or fewer syllables per line.) Bashō developed a new poetic form called* haibun*: a hybrid that alternates between prose and haiku and tells a story about one's travels. His most famous haibun,* Narrow Road to the Interior, *is about a 1,200-mile journey he made in May 1689.*

Here is a simple haiku from that book:

Still alive I am,
At the end of a long dream on my journey.
Fall of an autumn day.

♦

Tonight, as you settle into stillness, picture a ginkgo tree, perhaps with the glowing yellow leaves of autumn. As you close your eyes, imagine its leaves silently dropping in the night, leaving a thick carpet of yellow on the ground below.

Know that, like a ginkgo tree, you are singular.

You, too, are resilient.

You grow and change.

You survive hard times and complete long journeys.

Speak the poet's words aloud, maybe in a whisper: "Still alive I am, at the end of a long dream on my journey."

Still alive I am.

Still alive I am.

This can be your mantra tonight.

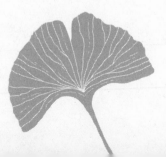

II

ELEPHANT

WHICH FORGETS ITSELF IN ITS GREATNESS

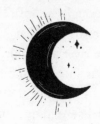

The Okavango Delta (in Botswana), one of the world's largest wetlands, appears on the UNESCO World Heritage list and is one of the seven natural wonders of Africa. Each year, water spreads over the delta when the Okavango River floods, drawing animals from all over the region. The delta boasts the largest remaining elephant population in the world, numbering more than 125,000. There are also lions, zebras, leopards, cheetahs, and more birds than can be counted—almost five hundred bird species have been documented in that area.

There are rhinoceroses there too, but their location is hidden due to their endangered status.

I was in southern Africa about twelve years ago on business, and before our work began, my team and I went to Botswana for a safari in the Okavango Delta. One day, we explored the delta by canoe. Our Botswanan guides gave us space to stop paddling, take pictures, and just sit in the stillness on the loop through the area. There was little sound except for the call of birds and that which my oars made, lightly splashing in the river alongside in my boat. Rounding a turn, though, I was shocked to find myself only ten or fifteen feet from a mother elephant and her baby crossing the water ahead of me. I slowed my canoe and froze. A few moments later, one of the guides glided up beside me.

"Oh," he said. "Oh."

I nodded.

We waited, in silence, and watched as the mother patiently taught the baby to cross the water. The mama elephant stood and waited for the baby to make its way toward the riverbank. But when her child seemed flustered or stuck, the mother would step around in front and take a few steps, modeling what it looked like to move in the water. She would then step back and wait. The baby took a step, and then another. Then it stood still again.

"Teaching her," the guide whispered. "Teaching her to do it."

We watched for what seemed like an hour, but I have no idea how long we were there. In the end, the baby garnered her confidence, walked forward, and approached the bank on the other side. Again, the mother watched and waited to see what her child would do. The baby put one foot, gingerly, up on the grassy slope but pulled it back. More quiet. More stillness. The baby tried again, its foot slipping back.

After what seemed like another delicious hour, the mother elephant gently touched the baby's rump with her trunk. The baby tried to climb again but slipped this time, getting dunked in the water. The mother stood still as the baby awkwardly stood to its feet again. She then nudged her baby between her back legs with her trunk. The baby scampered up onto the bank.

Two weeks later, at an airport souvenir shop in Johannesburg, South Africa, before flying home, I bought two small elephant figurines carved in dark ebony. I wanted to capture that magical experience, somehow take it back home with me. I keep them on my desk now, and sometimes I pick them up and examine them, letting my imagination take me back to the delta. Their trunks are raised, and I imagine they are the mother and the baby I watched as they made their way across the river. It still seems like a dream. Was I ever really that close to elephants in the wild?

My experience in Botswana led me into learning much more about these creatures than I had known before. I learned, for example, that there are three elephant species: Asian, African savanna, and African forest elephants. In the wild, Asian elephants can live up to eighty years; African elephants tend to live sixty or seventy years. African elephants have larger ears, and their skin is more wrinkled than Asian elephants. Their distinctive ears and skin help keep them cooler—when they flap their ears, blood vessels on the back of their ears help heat escape, and the natural wrinkles in their skin help them retain moisture. Elephants' other trademark physical feature, their trunks, also helps keep them cool. The fusion of its nose and upper lip, an elephant's trunk has more than four hundred thousand muscles, can lift more than four hundred pounds, and has enough fine motor control to pick up small objects—and, of course, elephants use it to spray water on themselves.

They also use their trunks to communicate, both by making sounds and by signaling with them as body language. With their close family bonds and social networks, elephants can recognize the sounds (snorts, barks, rumbles) made by family members and know when a call is coming from a stranger. They also make "seismic" sounds, or "infrasounds," ones too low to be audible to the human ear. These sounds carry over long distances; they can actually travel as far as thirty miles through the ground. Other elephants receive these messages through the sensitive skin of their trunks and feet.

It's no secret that they're smart; elephants are among the most intelligent creatures on earth. They're self-aware and one of the only animals able to recognize themselves in a mirror. They are also compassionate and emotionally complex. Like us, when someone they love dies, they grieve.

The late Lawrence Anthony, author of the book *The Elephant Whisperer*, was a conservationist with a storied history of befriending, caring for, and rescuing animals. After US-led coalition forces invaded Baghdad in 2003, it was Anthony who traveled to Iraq from his home in South Africa to save the animals of the Baghdad Zoo. He was one of the first civilians to enter Baghdad after the invasion, and despite the danger of entering a war zone, he was quoted as saying, "I couldn't stand the thought of the animals dying in their cages. . . . So I thought, I'll just go. I went there for the animals."

Anthony is most famous for the relationships he had with elephants, in particular a herd whose lives he saved and protected in his native South Africa. In *The Elephant Whisperer*, Anthony calls elephants "the largest and noblest of the land creatures" and details the lessons elephants taught him about parenting, unconditional love, and dignity. Anthony died in 2012, and his family reports that a group of the elephants visited his home after his death and stood outside for two days in silent vigil. One of Anthony's sons has said that the elephants have continued the memorial for several years, traveling more than twelve hours to pay their respects to their deceased friend.

It isn't just how close I was to the elephants that continues to move me to this day. Nor was it the sense of real awe that emanated from the guide sitting still in his canoe beside me, despite the fact that he lived in the delta and had seen elephants in the wild many times before that day.

The experience leaves me with a gentle, reverent feeling, akin to the sense I've had when walking in the evening at twilight, before shades are drawn, happening to see into someone else's well-lit home. Seeing people in my neighborhood just going about their lives, alone or in the company of others, evokes a similar sense. Maybe someone is simply unloading a dishwasher or reading to a child or folding up a blanket or paging through a stack of mail. Families are just doing their everyday, ordinary acts whether anyone is watching or not.

Walking by and glancing in a neighbor's window, I get to bear witness to their ordinary and yet sacred lives. I get to see our common dignity and to appreciate that each and every one of us is just living one day after another, step by step.

◆

Too-qua-stee, a member of the Cherokee Nation, was an academic, attorney, political writer, and poet who was born in 1829.

Educated in Native American boarding schools as a child, he graduated with honors from Dartmouth College in 1861. Also known as DeWitt Clinton Duncan, Too-qua-stee studied Cherokee history and linguistics, and he contributed to both Cherokee and English literary publications.

Read these lines from Too-qua-stee's poem "Dignity":

True dignity is like a summer tree.
Beneath whose shade both beast, and bird, and bee,
When by the heated skies oppressed, may come,
And feel, in its magnificence, at home;
Or rather like a mountain which forgets
Itself in its own greatness, and so lets
Vast armies fuss and fight upon its sides,
While high in clouds its peaceful summit hides,
And from the voiceless crest of glistening snow,
Pours trickling fatness on the fields below;
Repellant force, that daunts obtrusive wrong,
And woos the timid steps of right along.

◆

Quiet your mind for a moment and find your breath. Open your heart to the knowledge that it's only an illusion that creatures like elephants and humans are so different, so separate. Think of the ways we are connected, how we experience our lives in similar ways. Elephants communicate with each other, teach their young, and even experience heartache, just as we do. They live their lives with dignity.

Tonight, as you settle in for sleep, think of times you took "timid steps" to do what is right.

Think of a time when you taught something useful to someone else, perhaps to a child in your life. When have you modeled a good way to live? Maybe you did something small, like holding the door or offering up your seat to a stranger. You affirmed someone else's dignity and put others first.

Look back on Too-qua-stee's poem. How might dignity be like "a summer tree"? How is it "a mountain that forgets"?

Remember that you are a person who is worthy of honor and respect.

You have the right to live with dignity as you, step by step, go about your own ordinary, extraordinary life.

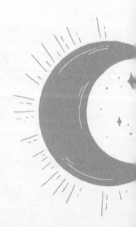

12
THE KADUPUL

A PRAYER LIKE INCENSE

My husband's grandmother lives in a retirement home in the gentle, rolling hills of eastern Pennsylvania. At one hundred, she's in fairly good health, and her memory is strong. The most significant obstacle she lives with is that after years of declining eyesight, she is now legally blind.

The last time we visited her in person, two of my children and I chatted with her in her room. On her walls hang photographs, prints, paintings, and a cross-stitch sampler. The sampler and one of the paintings are original works, created just for her many years ago by her former Sunday school students. They are the work of amateur artists, possibly children. The stitches in the cross-stitch aren't uniform, and the perspective and shadows aren't quite right in the painting. And Grandma loves them. She tells us the stories behind these and other pictures on the wall, gesturing toward them. She no longer can see them with her eyes, but she sees with the vision that is her memory.

"You see the photograph above my bed?" she asks, her head slightly bowed. Over the past few years, she has begun sitting that way much of the time: head lowered as though she is about to say grace. Above her bed hangs an old photograph, in sepia tones, of three women threshing wheat. Its mahogany oval frame shines.

"I loved it when I first saw it, but I didn't want Jonas to buy it for me," she explains. "It was too expensive. But he went back to the antique shop on his own and surprised me."

She giggles, remembering the romantic gesture. She has been widowed twice; Jonas, her second husband, passed away several years ago. Jonas was a chicken farmer, given to wearing suspenders, and the great-grandpa my children knew. A conscientious objector, he worked for the National Park Service as a young man during World War II building fences and clearing land. Even as a very old man, his hands were large and strong, his words humble, and his voice gentle with love. Grandma tells us what drew her to the picture: the grace of the women in their long skirts, the beauty of the composition, and the way it honors hard work.

Later, she tells us how she is spending her days now. She begins the day in prayer by reciting Psalm 23, then goes to breakfast with the help of an orderly named Pete. She tells us that they talk baseball together and that he's always ready with a joke.

"He's probably my best friend!" she says, and then she erupts into laughter. She seems surprised that she has just described him this way. Most of her friends have passed away, but she has Pete. She sits quietly for a few moments, shaking her head. "He's good company," she says.

Often, she listens to audiobooks—histories and biographies are her favorites. And sometimes she sings hymns, alone, in her room. At the end of the day, she tells us, before going to bed, she recites Psalm 23 again and prays the Lord's Prayer. She says she prays for everyone in the family, speaking our names aloud, one by one. These private acts of worship, these prayers faithfully uttered night after night, are spoken in the dark and not seen or heard by anyone but God.

Sitting on the edge of her bed, I think of a video I came across recently that captured an exotic flower blooming in time-lapse. The flower is one of the rarest in the world: the Kadupul. Variously called Queen of the Night, Flower from the Heaven, and Beauty under the Moon, the Kadupul only rarely blooms and only in certain months of the year and on nights when there is a full moon. On those occasions, it opens for a few hours and wilts before dawn. It's literally priceless because once picked, it withers away; it can never be sold in a store. In China, people use the name of the flower to describe someone who has a fleeting moment of fame. We Americans might call someone's short-lived success a "flash in the pan," but in China, they reference the Kadupul.

The Kadupul resembles a water lily with its bright white petals and rose-colored stem, but when it opens completely, it looks more like a burst of light with long spiky outer petals and delicate yellow filament. Like an orchid, it grows in the forks of trees. Its thick leaves are long and have scalloped edges. The flower is loved not only for its beauty but for the deeply calming fragrance that it emits. Soothing and distinct, its fragrance has been called the "midnight miracle." In parts of Southeast Asia, some people believe that prayers are more likely to be answered on the nights when the Kadupul blooms. The only way to see it in person is to visit its home in the tropical rain forest—at just the right time in one of those months and only on one of those full moon nights.

Sometimes at night, I think of Grandma sitting alone in her room in the dark speaking my name and those of my children. Psalm 141:2 reads, "May my prayer be set before you like incense; may the lifting up of my hands be like the evening sacrifice" (NIV). I imagine her quiet, trusting prayers rising like incense or like the fragrance of the Kadupul to God: a beautiful, private act of worship.

Knowing she is there praying for me, I'm blanketed in a sense of deep calm.

◆

*Rabindranath Tagore, sometimes called "the Bard of Bengal,"
was a poet, philosopher, composer, and painter. (Bengal is now
divided between the Indian state of West Bengal and the People's
Republic of Bangladesh.) A close friend of Gandhi, he also par-
ticipated in the Indian nationalist movement. In 1913, Tagore
became the first non-European writer to win the Nobel Prize in
Literature. The committee said he received the honor "because
of his profoundly sensitive, fresh and beautiful verse, by which,
with consummate skill, he has made his poetic thought, expressed
in his own English words, a part of the literature of the West."*

Read these lines excerpted from "The Gift," a poem by Tagore:

*Whatever gifts are in my power to give you,
Be they flowers,
Be they gems for your neck
How can they please you
If in time they must surely wither,
Crack,
Lose luster?*

*Rather,
When you have leisure,
Wander idly through my garden in spring
And let an unknown, hidden flower's scent startle you*

Into sudden wondering—
Let that displaced moment
Be my gift.

♦

The poet wishes to give a gift to someone he loves but hesitates, knowing that all things, as he writes elsewhere in the poem, "turn into dust." He decides, then, to give his lover the gift of a beautiful "displaced moment": the surprise scent of a flower in his garden.

As you prepare for sleep, consider what the Kadupul and the "hidden flower" in Tagore's poem have in common. They are not cut or picked, but they are enjoyed right where they grow and left untouched. The person who experiences their beauty can't control, contain, or own them but simply enjoys them in the present moment.

Take a few deep breaths, breathing out longer than you breathe in. Allow your memory to call forth an evocative scent. See where it takes you.

Call to mind the face of someone you love, and practice a loving-kindness meditation for them. Perhaps you associate a scent with this person: the perfume or cologne they wear, a candle they burn in their home, the flowers in their garden, or something else. Allow your memory to call it forth.

Ask God to keep that person safe, happy, healthy, and living with ease. You could use the following simple phrases as you hold them in your thoughts:

May you be safe.
May you be happy.
May you be healthy.
May you live with ease.

As you prepare for sleep, imagine your prayers and intentions rising up to heaven like the fragrance of a beautiful flower.

13
PATTERNS

THE INFINITE COMPLEXITY OF CREATED THINGS

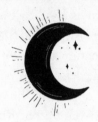

Imagine that you're standing at the kitchen counter preparing a head of broccoli to serve for dinner. Cutting the florets from the stalk, you notice that each of the smaller parts on your cutting board resembles the whole. Cut one smaller and, well, the same is true. Pull off a tiny, fresh shoot, and you have a minuscule version of that floret, a perfect miniature of the whole head. The shape just keeps repeating itself, over and over, as it's rendered smaller and smaller.

Or imagine walking through the forest and stopping to look at a fern growing at the base of a tree. You notice that its individual leaves resemble the frond; they're tiny copies of the whole branch.

Or think of the shape of lightning, a jagged stick of fire in the night sky. Each branch is a replica of the whole bolt.

All these things—the broccoli, the fern, and the lightning bolt—are known as "fractals." The word *fractal* was coined in 1975 by Benoit Mandelbrot, a mathematician born in what used to be known as Eastern Europe and who spent most of his adulthood in the United States. Mandelbrot saw patterns and order in nature and spent his career exploring and describing them. He defined *fractals* as shapes that, when divided, create smaller replicas of the whole. The term is an adaptation of the Latin word *fractus*, meaning "fragmented or broken." Fractals are infinitely complex, infinitely repeating, like a Russian nesting doll.

Mandelbrot, describing his upbringing and education, said,

For the first and second grades I was tutored privately by the husband of an aunt, because my mother, a doctor, was scared of epidemics and kept me away from school. That uncle was an intellectual who despised rote learning, including even the alphabet and the table of multiplication: both mildly trouble me to this day. However, he trained my memory and my mind in an independent and creative way through extensive reading. Most of my time was spent playing chess, reading maps and learning how to open my eyes to everything around me. Certainly, these experiences did not harm, probably even helped the geometric intuition which has been my most important intellectual tool.

So due to the way his memory was trained, and thanks to the fact that he was taught to open his eyes to everything around him, we now understand the approximate order of the natural world in ways we wouldn't have otherwise. Mandelbrot's breakthrough book *The Fractal Geometry of Nature* finally legitimized his work, when, for many years previously, people considered his theories a bit, you could say, "off."

Fractals reveal their inner workings and the way they were formed. Trees, for instance, grow by repetitive branching. The main branches keep repeating themselves in the smaller branches and limbs, illustrating "self-similarity": a pattern that repeats itself at different scales. Hurricanes, in their spiral shape, are infinitely repeating fractals that also clearly demonstrate how they're made. Abstract or mathematical fractals can be generated by a computer by calculating the same equations over and over and over again.

The Fibonacci sequence is a mathematical fractal. Also known as the golden spiral, golden ratio, or the divine proportion, it often appears, as if by miracle, in the natural world.

It is the series of numbers in which every *next* number in the sequence is the sum of the two numbers that came just before it: 0, 1, 1, 2, 3, 5, 8, 13, 21, 34, and so on. (If you, like me, don't consider math your very best subject, just scoot back for a sec and look at that pattern. If I can see it, I promise you can too: 0 + 1 = **1**, 1 + 1 = **2**, 2 + 1 = **3**, and so on.) What's more, the stunning thing is that you can *see* that golden ratio in the pattern of seeds on the face of sunflower and in the exacting, curved spiral of a nautilus shell and occurring in countless other places. (I mentioned broccoli—the everyday kind you find in the produce section—above as an example of an approximate fractal. If you've ever seen Romanesco broccoli, with its spiky, spiraling buds, you see a truer example of a fractal. Each bud on a head of Romanesco broccoli is composed of a series of smaller buds all arranged in perfect spirals that repeat over and over again.)

It's bizarre, but our bodies are also fractals, following a sequence of 1, 2, 3, 5, and so on. It's evident from a quick look in the mirror (we have one nose, two eyes, three parts of each limb, and five fingers on each hand and foot), but human DNA and the rhythm of a healthy heartbeat also follow a fractal pattern. Our lungs, too, are natural fractal organs. From the Fractal Foundation, "The lungs share the same branching pattern as the trees. And it is for good reason! Both the trees and lungs have evolved to serve a similar function—respiration. Since they perform a similar function, it should not be surprising that they share a similar structure. This common concept in science is known as the Structure-Function Relationship. Many of the fractals in biological systems . . . have evolved their structures in order to perform extraordinary functions. In the case of Lungs and Trees, they both breathe."

Fractals aren't the only mysterious, intriguing, and surprisingly orderly patterns we find in nature, of course. There are symmetries, spots and stripes, and the wonderfully named "meanders," which describe both the way a snake moves and how a river twists and turns through a landscape. What about the ripple pattern that wind leaves on water or sand, the geometry of honeycombs, tessellations, and more? Time is a pattern and full of patterns; some physicists even argue that time *itself* is a fractal. Language is full of patterns: To make nouns plural, we usually add an *s*. We repeat end sounds of words to create rhymes. In our dedication to pattern, we even look for and produce palindromes—words and sentences that read the same backward and forward. There are simple ones like "mom" and "madam" and trickier ones like "Never odd or even!" and "Was it a cat I saw?"

Patterns are everywhere, bringing rhythm, order, beauty, and whimsy to our lives.

Viola Spolin is known as the "Mother of Improv." Her book *Improvisation for the Theater*, published in 1963, is still considered an essential theater text. The actress and director created exercises—or "theater games"—for actors, helping them become playful and open in their work. In some of her games, actors speak in gibberish; in others, they sing their lines, and many involve physical games that get actors moving in full and fluid ways. Spolin writes that theater games free the student "for the flowing, endless pattern of stage behavior."

I'm not an actor, but I love Spolin's book for its celebration of the creative process. I read *Improvisation for the Theater* during graduate school to spark ideas for the academic papers I was writing. I paged through it as a young mother looking for inventive ways to interact with my kids. I still look at it from time to time, hungry for her optimistic, buoyant wisdom. Reading Spolin's book is a creative palate cleanser for me. "Creativity is an attitude, a way of looking at something, a way of questioning, perhaps a way of life—it may well be found on paths we have not yet traveled," she writes. "Creativity is curiosity, joy, and communion."

One theater game is called "Patterns." In it, acting students stand at the edges of a rehearsal space, and one student begins the game by walking to the center of the room and striking—and then holding—a pose. Then, one by one, all of the others come to the center, mirroring or building off that first student's stance until everyone joins. No one speaks or moves quickly as they create something unique and new from their individual selves. The living sculpture created by the actors' repetitive branching is a pattern that tells the story of how it was made, and it seems like an approximate metaphor for the infinite patterns of fractals in nature. Fractals tell the story of the processes that create them too—like the spirals of hurricanes or the branching patterns of trees. Created by the repetition of a simple process, they seem, somehow, infused with joy.

◆

Read this prayer from the Book of Common Prayer: "Almighty and everlasting God, you made the universe with all its marvelous order, its atoms, worlds, and galaxies, and the infinite complexity of living creatures: Grant that, as we probe the mysteries of your creation, we may come to know you more truly. Amen."

◆

Tonight, before you drift off to sleep, practice a "full-body scan" exercise. This practice can help you tune in to and connect with your physical self. In it, you notice anything you're feeling—sensations, itches, warmth, aches, relaxation, tingling—and you notice them without judgment.

If this is the first time you have practiced a body-scan meditation, here are a few tips:

- *Begin by focusing your attention on the top of your head and slowly move down to your toes.*

- *Breathe deeply, letting your abdomen expand and contract with each breath.*
- *Focus on each part of your body, just lingering there for a moment.*
- *Don't worry about any discomfort or sensations you might be feeling. Just recognize what you feel and softly name it, such as "relaxed shoulders," "expanding chest," "warmth around my stomach," or "tightness in my calves." Then slowly move down to the next area of your body.*

When you reach the bottom of your feet, breathe a long breath out. Think about the infinite complexity of your human form, of the world of nature, and of the way your life interacts and branches off from the lives of other people.

Think about the fact that the way your imagination, perspective, and creativity were formed is reflected in who you are today.

You are, in your own way, a fractal: your life tells the story of the processes that have made you exactly who you are.

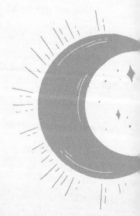

14

RED-WINGED BLACKBIRDS

THE HEART FINDS ITS MORNING AND IS REFRESHED

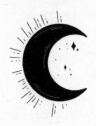

Red-winged blackbirds are one of the most abundant birds in North America. The males are easily identifiable by their glossy black feathers and the red and yellow patches on their shoulders, while the females—sometimes mistaken for sparrows—are dark brown, are streaked with tan stripes, and have a fine mist of yellow around their bills. I hear their chirps ("check, check") and songs ("konk-la-*reeee*") almost every day in spring and summer on walks around the marshy lake near my house. We've talked about murmurations of starlings and glitterings of hummingbirds and even an implausibility of gnus, so you might have guessed there are playful words for a flock of red-winged blackbirds too. A group of blackbirds is known as a *cloud*, a *cluster*, or a *merle*. Or you can just call it a flock. Red-winged blackbirds roost in flocks all year long. In summer, they're in smaller numbers in wetland areas; in winter, they join flocks that can be as large as several million birds.

Male red-winged blackbirds are famously aggressive toward suspected predators, including human passersby, when they sense that their nests are threatened. I've hurried away from the edge of the lake in spring many times when a red-winged blackbird has given me a stern chirp from his perch. And more than once, I've witnessed a redwing as though he's an extra in Hitchcock's thriller *The Birds*, dive-bombing someone who has ignored his warning.

You can't blame him for being stressed: a male red-winged blackbird has as many as fifteen nests in his territory to guard. These nests, built exclusively by female redwings over the course of three to six days, are lined with dried mud and grass, are shaped like cups, and woven with grass, leaves, and other vegetation. They're about four to seven inches across and just about as deep, hidden among the reeds and cattails. Each female lays three to five eggs every season, pale blue-green with dark spots that mostly appear around the larger end of the egg. Given that these birds are polygynous, females often lay clutches of mixed paternity. So one male can be looking out for as many as sixty nestlings a season—or even more—and not all of them will be his biological offspring.

Redwings nest in what are called "loose colonies," allowing for more adult birds to be present and alert to threats from predators like hawks and raccoons as well as from the parasitic cowbird, who, when a female redwing has momentarily left the nest, hurries to lay her eggs there. At the cowbird's approach, a male redwing might either sound an alarm, drawing the female back to her nest, or swoop in to dissuade her. Some studies have shown that redwings and other species, such as yellow warblers, communicate with each other to warn of a visit from a brood parasite like the cowbird.

Friendship and *chosen family* might not be the first concepts to come to mind when you think about birds. Yet these facts—that the male redwing accepts and cares for nestlings not his own and that birds live in community with other species—echo committed relationships in human life that nurture and sustain us, including those not bound by biology, like marriage or the adoption or a child. I've used the term *chosen family* many times over the years to describe a few special people in my life. The term *chosen family* was coined at least one hundred years ago in the LGBTQ+ community; chosen families of friends set up households together after being estranged from or rejected by their families of origin. For any of us who have lived far away from our families, haven't felt accepted or celebrated by them, or otherwise have unmet familial needs, chosen family is one of life's most precious gifts. Human beings (well, most creatures too) *need* social support. When we've felt rejected or misunderstood by the families we first knew, or when we feel forced into old, uncomfortable roles when we are with them, chosen family can be redemptive.

In a scholarly article about chosen family in the context of the LGBTQ+ community and mental health, anthropologist Nina Jackson Levin and her coauthors write, "Chosen family implies an alternative formulation that subverts, rejects, or overrides . . . an American paradigm of kinship." One of the subjects in the study describes her experience with chosen family, saying, "To me there's a difference between [chosen family] and friends because friends are people that you enjoy being around, but chosen family is more . . . who comes to my house and eats with me? Who do I cook for, you know? I think 'who do I cook for' is a good easy way to tell if somebody's part of my chosen family or just a friend."

An editor friend tells me about plans for the upcoming holiday, saying that his kids are coming to town. "Well, they're not *my* kids," he says, fumbling for the right words. "I mean, my wife didn't give birth to them, and we didn't legally adopt them, but they're our kids. Have been for twenty years."

"Chosen family," I say.

That his kids are coming to town for the holidays points out another element that seems critical in chosen families: celebrating rituals, especially around meals, together. In the study mentioned above, the authors underscore the importance of cooking for and eating with others: "In each of these cases, gathering around food served as a foundation for establishing consistent, nourishing rituals. While meals were often discussed as practices for celebrating chosen family, feeding each other was also described as a form of mental and physical health care."

When not out playing the role of "knight of the prairie"—a nickname given to the male redwing owing to the way he valiantly defends his community—he is out feeding and finding food for his nestlings. He often travels as far as fifty miles from his territory before coming back home to the nests. Like the redwing, we feed and nourish our friends. Chosen family is about intentionality, commitment, and deep and mutual support.

♦

Kahlil Gibran was a Lebanese American writer. He is best known as the author of The Prophet, *one of the best-selling books of all time; it has remained in print since its publication in 1923. The book is a series of parables on topics including prayer, beauty, religion, and yes, friendship.*

Read these lines from the prose poem "On Friendship" from
The Prophet:

Your friend is your needs answered.
He is your field which you sow with love and reap with
thanksgiving.
And he is your board and your fireside.
For you come to him with your hunger, and you seek
him for peace.
And let there be no purpose in friendship save the deep-
ening of the spirit.
For love that seeks aught but the disclosure of its own
mystery is not love but a net cast forth: and only the
unprofitable is caught.
And let your best be for your friend.
If he must know the ebb of your tide, let him know its
flood also.
For what is your friend that you should seek him with
hours to kill?
Seek him always with hours to live.
For it is his to fill your need but not your emptiness.
And in the sweetness of friendship let there be laughter,
and sharing of pleasures.
For in the dew of little things the heart finds its morn-
ing and is refreshed.

◆

Tonight, bring to mind the face of a friend who is "chosen family" for you. Close your eyes and allow your mind's eye to fill in details about your friend.

Think specifically about this person. Imagine their hair color, the way their eyes look when they smile. What does this person's favorite shirt look like? How do they hold their coffee cup? What makes them laugh?

Does your memory bring you a detail you didn't even know you had noticed about your friend? Take a moment just to be present with that person in your mind.

Remember the way you came into each other's lives. Did you meet at school? At work? By chance?

In what ways is this friend, as Gibran says, "your needs answered"?

How does this friend deepen your spirit?

When has this friend helped your heart "find its morning" or be refreshed?

Say a word of thanks that this person is in your life.

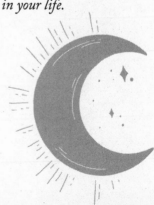

15

MURMURATIONS

BY ANALOGY, THEIR AUTHOR IS SEEN

The book of Wisdom is considered by some Christians an apocryphal work—not part of the official scriptural canon. It is, however, part of the Catholic Bible. Grouped with other Wisdom books, including Psalms, Proverbs, and Ecclesiastes, Wisdom is similarly rich and poetic. In it, the quality of wisdom is personified, and she is a woman. Wisdom is a "kindly spirit," is "resplendent and unfading," and "hastens to make herself known to those who desire her" (Wisdom 1:6; 6:12; 6:13 NABRE).

My favorite part of the book is chapter 13, in which the author (thought by some to be wise King Solomon) makes a bold and startling claim: "From the greatness and the beauty of created things," he writes, "their original author, by analogy, is seen" (Wisdom 13:5 NABRE). In other words, Wisdom tells us that the beautiful things we observe in nature are actually *metaphors for God*.

That idea brings to mind one of nature's most mysterious and striking visions: starling murmurations. I've seen flocks of starlings rising and falling at twilight above farmland in rural Illinois, and I've watched clips of this phenomenon dozens of times online. But whether I'm seeing a murmuration live or viewing a video of this aerial ballet, I feel spellbound. And I wonder, In what ways might a murmuration be a metaphor for the Divine?

A single starling is a small, humble-looking black bird. But when starlings gather at dusk—by the hundreds and even thousands—whirling and swooping in coordinated flight, they become what seems to be one massive creature. The birds darken the sky like plumes of thick smoke, disperse and disappear, then come together again, diving in synchronized patterns. They murmur and hum, the sounds of their thousands of beating wings like ocean waves. Watching a murmuration, you see them form the spiral shape of a tornado until that funnel cloud melts into a great sea creature that rises up, only to morph suddenly into the shape of something like a swan before they dissipate and shape-shift again.

Unlike hummingbirds, starlings are sociable birds, and they flock together in large groups. The term *murmuration* can be used to describe both their flocks and their mesmerizing flight formations. Researchers have theories about this behavior, although there are always still questions. Does murmurating keep them warm? Are they hunting? Is it a way to communicate with each other about food sources? Most agree that when starlings flock like this, it's antipredatory behavior, a coordinated attempt to outwit the hawks and falcons—birds whose eyesight is four to eight times sharper than ours—who prey on them.

Fish, bees, bats, and many other creatures also swarm and cluster to protect themselves when they are threatened. Instead of appearing as one vulnerable individual, they blur the line between "individual" and "group," creating the illusion of power by joining together. United, they become loud, large, and confusing to the creatures that would harm them. Human beings do this too—we gather and organize ourselves and move together as one when we feel like our convictions or our liberties or our lives are under attack.

John Updike, in his poem "The Great Scarf of Birds," describes murmurations as iron filings being manipulated by a magnet, "a lady's scarf," and an ink stain. In that poem, Updike reflects on starlings' synchronized movement and wonders whether one of the birds is directing all the others in their formation because it was either "prompted by accident" or had the "will to lead." Updike wrote his poem in the early 1960s. About thirty years earlier, an ornithologist had proposed that starlings used telepathy, or "thought-transference," to coordinate their movements! Since then, much more has been learned about how starlings orchestrate their murmurations.

We now know that the birds can flock like this without crashing into one other because of something called "rapid coordinated collective response." In a flock of thousands of birds, while individuals can't keep track of the motion or behavior of every other bird, they *can* pay attention to, respond to, and replicate the location, direction, and speed of the six or seven birds closest to them. All the small groupings of starlings within a murmuration respond quickly to one another, and their behavior spreads, in waves, through the entire group.

Birds also "see faster" than we do; they see at more than twice the speed of the human eye. In our (and birds') eyes, light-sensitive cells react to light, send a signal to the brain, and then refresh in order to receive the next visual signal. Birds' eyes do this very, very quickly, allowing them to snap up flying insects and quickly avoid moving obstacles like tree branches blowing in the wind or other birds in flight. Because of this ultrarapid vision, as it's called, it's as though they can see life in slow motion.

So in what ways could a murmuration be a metaphor for the Divine? Does it tell us that God's vision is different from ours? That the Spirit is creative and ever in motion, able to make huge, beautiful things from tiny, humble parts? Do murmurations show us that God flies? Swoops? Gathers? That God's Spirit murmurs?

Or perhaps murmurations are metaphors for Christ or for the church. St. Paul describes the church as the body of Christ and as one body with many members: "For just as the body is one and has many members, and all the members of the body, though many, are one body, so it is with Christ. . . . Indeed, the body does not consist of one member but of many. . . . If one member suffers, all suffer together with it; if one member is honored, all rejoice together with it. Now you are the body of Christ and individually members of it" (1 Corinthians 12:12, 14, 26–27). What a surprising set of images, so laden not only with mystery but with assertions about how indispensable we are to one another.

Or we could consider murmurations a metaphor for the Trinity—for what Franciscan author Richard Rohr calls "the Divine dance." Like a murmuration of birds, the Christian doctrine of the Trinity holds that there is one God, who is mystically composed of three divine "persons"— sometimes called the Father, Son, and Holy Spirit or the Creator, Redeemer, and Sustainer. Rohr describes the mutuality, communication, and enjoyment he believes define the Trinity. He says that the Trinity reveals, simply put, that God *is* relationship. To say that a murmuration is about rapid, coordinated, collective response is to point to its mutuality too. I can't help imagining the starlings are having fun together in flight; Rohr says that God is "Flow," and that Flow is love.

All of these ideas capture my imagination. Yet I feel most at home with the idea that starling murmurations serve to remind us that God is a mystery and impossible to capture in words. That is, unlike so many topics in this book—dandelions, ginkgos, and honey—murmurations force us to rely on the approximate language of metaphor when we attempt to understand them.

Updike, in his poem, conjures up images of iron filings and a woman's scarf tossed over a chair. I see them as dark plumes of smoke and say that they shape-shift into sea creatures and swans. It's like that, too, when we try to talk about our experiences and conceptions of God. We fumble around and reach for figurative language. The way I see, experience, and describe the Divine is very different from the way you do.

Starling murmurations, like the Divine, are steeped in otherness. They rely on relationship. They are a mystery to us. They see faster than we do, and they experience time in a wholly different way than we do. Murmurations of starlings sometimes appear to us, just like God does, from seemingly out of nowhere—the visions taking us by surprise, sometimes just as night is falling.

♦

Julian of Norwich was an English mystic in the Middle Ages. When she was thirty years old, she became very ill. For two days, lying on her deathbed after last rites had been administered, Julian saw visions, which she would later call "showings," of Christ. She miraculously recovered from her illness, and twenty years later, after reflecting on their meaning, she recorded these visions. Her book Revelations of Divine Love *is the earliest surviving book written in English by a woman. The most famous quotation from the book is spoken by Christ to Julian; Christ assures her that "all shall be well, and all shall be well, and all manner of thing shall be well."*

Read these words of Julian's: "God All-Power is our natural Father, and God All-Wisdom is our natural Mother, supported by the boundless Love and Goodness of the Holy Spirit. All One God. He is our true partner in this weaving and joining. . . . He says, 'I love you and you love me, and our love will never be broken in two.'"

God All-Wisdom, whom Julian calls our "natural Mother," hurries to us when we seek her. Do you seek wisdom or discernment in some part of your life? Remember that God is with you in the "weaving and joining" that is your life.

♦

Tonight, as you drift off to sleep, try to imagine a great, swooping cloud of starlings shape-shifting in the sky. What forms do you see? What images does your psyche, your spirit, bring forth as you watch them with your mind's eye?

Imagine the starlings are trying to tell you something about the goodness and love of Mother God.

Thank God for her wisdom.

After you close your eyes tonight, speak these words, silently, to whomever you understand God to be: "Our love will never be broken in two."

16

REDWOODS

TO BATHE IN HER AS IN A SEA

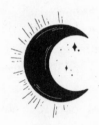

Entering Muir Woods feels like entering a cathedral; it is a holy place. The electric green of ferns, their fronds perfect fractals, borders the pathway. Jade-green moss and lichen artfully dot tree trunks. Sunlight breaks through the canopy as through a stained glass window, lighting the deep, rich brown of the massive trunks that vault up into the sky. You feel reverent looking up and around. Anne Lamott has famously said that while she doesn't need to understand complex theology or the Trinity, she does want to give her life to "whoever came up with redwood trees."

Named for John Muir, a Scottish American naturalist, environmental activist, and author known as the "Father of the National Parks" in the United States, Muir Woods is part of the Golden Gate National Recreation Area twelve miles north of San Francisco. It contains 240 acres of old-growth redwoods, most of which are between 600 and 800 years old; the oldest one there is about 1,200 years old. Redwoods have been in California for at least twenty million years; by comparison, early *Homo sapiens*, who looked much like we do and had brains the same size as ours, have only been around since about 130,000 years ago.

The silence my husband and I keep when we are there, in the presence of these ancient redwoods, is restorative. Just the day before, we'd said goodbye to our young adult son, our eldest, having helped him settle into his apartment in San Francisco. I know he made a good choice going to live there. It is all right and good, but this was the first time one of my children moved out of state. Like so many other parental firsts, I felt out of my depth, uncertain, and a little shaky.

After we said goodbye, my husband at the wheel of our rental car, a text from my friend Cathleen lit up my phone. She had seen the pictures of our trip that I'd posted online and asked how I was doing, knowing it was hard to move my son so far from home.

"Feeling pretty tender," I admitted. "But tomorrow—Muir Woods!"

"Lean into the trees," she answered. "They hold so much wisdom."

Her words were like an invitation, a blessing. Through the invisible network that connects us, her love nurtures me.

Climbing a steep hiking trail the next day, I silently repeat Cathleen's advice: *lean into the trees.* It keeps me present, right here and right now. Every so often, walking past one of the trees, I stop and press the palm of my hand on its trunk. The thick bark is rough and cool, and somehow, the tree seems to express a kind of consciousness. An intelligence. Do I discern a response to my touch, somehow, from deep within the tree? There is a wisdom about these trees. I wonder what they are telling me. That time goes on? That my roots are deep? That I will weather this particular time and the transitions to come? That my son is safe here? That they'll shelter him? Whatever their message, it feels deeply kind, and it quiets me.

In Japan, beginning in the 1980s, the Ministry of Agriculture began promoting a practice called Shinrin-yoku, or "taking in the forest." Known as "forest bathing" in the United States, this practice means not just spending time in the woods but being truly present to the trees by using the senses: looking at the colors of leaves and pine needles; feeling the texture of bark, rocks, and leaves; smelling the scent of pine needles and wildflowers. Numerous studies have shown how this practice is good for not only our mental health but our general health as well. A study funded by the National

Institutes of Health in the United States says that Shinrin-yoku is now considered a "pivotal part of preventative health care and healing in Japanese medicine" and makes a case for medical and mental health providers in the United States including it in their care. The authors suggest that research points to "a plethora of positive health benefits for the human physiological and psychological systems," including benefits to immune system function as well as to the cardiovascular and respiratory systems and mental health.

Like other mindfulness practices, forest bathing isn't about judging or evaluating an experience. It's about using our senses and being present, focusing on what we see, hear, feel, smell, and taste right here, right now. It brings us back from worrying about the future or regretting the past; it heals us. And today, walking through Muir Woods with my new guidebook in hand, I experience that healing.

Looking up at a tree that's more than 250 feet tall, I consider that these trees come from seeds smaller than tomato seeds. And their root systems are surprisingly shallow, sometimes only about five or six feet deep. They garner their strength not by means of deep taproots but by extending their roots widely, up to one hundred feet from their trunks. They connect with the roots of other trees, forming a huge, mutual, braided root mass under the forest floor. They stand tall and stay strong because of each other. They're in community.

What's more, according to biologists including Suzanne Simard, whose TED talk on forests has been viewed millions of times, trees' intertwined roots do more than provide stability. Simard's research has shown that trees actually *communicate* with one another this way. She explains that they speak silently to one another by sending signals to each other via a web of fungi called a mycorrhizal network, which connects the roots of trees in a forest and creates a kind of central nervous system. She has described that network as being something like the internet—nearly every tree in the forest is connected and shares information, underground, with each other. Through the fungi that link trees with one another via their roots, trees share carbon, water, and nutrients with each other, sending what's most needed to the most vulnerable trees when they "call" for help. They even move nutrients such as nitrogen to other species of plants in the ecosystem. The forest, she reveals, is a place of community and mutual care.

High up on a hiking trail, I look down a steep ravine onto the rocky creek that cuts through Muir Woods. I learn in my guidebook that redwoods not only rely on rain to survive, but they "drink" the fog that comes off the Pacific Ocean, gaining sustenance from nutrients in the fog as well. I also discover that redwoods, like mangroves in the tropics, fight climate change by "sequestering" carbon. There are three main types of carbon sequestration, or the capture and storage of carbon that otherwise would remain in or be released into the atmosphere, causing global warming. These massive redwoods, practicing biologic carbon sequestration, capture more carbon dioxide than any other trees on earth. Muir Woods also supports the health of the planet by offering a safe habitat for coho salmon and other fish as well as for mountain lions. With bark that can be one-foot thick, the trees are protected from fire, insects, and disease.

In some parts of the forest, I observe a circle of trees around a bare spot, as if they were intentionally planted in a ring. I learn that these are called "family circles" and that the ring of trees is likely a group of clones of a long-dead tree. Instead of growing from seeds, this group sprouts from a "mother" tree. When a mother tree dies, new trees spring up in her circular footprint, each tree in the family circle carrying the mother's genetic material. Seeing these rings of trees gives me a reassuring sense of my own family legacy, the way it will continue after me, my children together, mutually caring for each other, connected in community.

At the end of the day, we reluctantly leave the woods.

"Feel better?" my husband asks as we get into the car.

I do. The redwoods have bathed me in comfort and have lifted my spirits with their age, beauty, and wisdom.

◆

John Burroughs was an American naturalist and author in the nineteenth century. Burroughs's writing was very popular during his lifetime, although he's far less well known than his famous friends Walt Whitman, Thomas Edison, Henry Ford, and John Muir.

Burroughs considered himself not a scientist but a literary naturalist who loved to write about his own relationship with the natural world. I connect with his words about how he approaches nature: "I am not always in sympathy with nature-study as pursued in the schools. . . . Such study is too cold, too special, too mechanical; it is likely to rub the bloom off Nature. . . . I myself have never made a dead set at studying Nature with note-book and field-glass in hand. I have rather visited with her. We have walked together or sat down together, and our intimacy grows with the seasons. . . . To absorb a thing is better than to learn it, and we absorb what we enjoy."

He goes on to say, "I go to Nature to be soothed and healed, and to have my senses put in tune once more. . . . I do not go to Nature to be taught. I go for enjoyment and companionship. I go to bathe in her as in a sea; I go to give my eyes and ears and all of my senses a free, clean field."

♦

Take three deep, soothing breaths. Try to breathe out longer than you inhale, perhaps breathing in through your nose for four seconds and then out for eight.

Let your body relax.

As you move toward sleep tonight, imagine you are walking in a deep forest.

What do you see?

What do you touch?

What do you feel?

What companionship or wisdom might the forest offer you?

Imagine now a "family circle" of redwoods: a ring of trees that have grown from a mother tree. In your mind, stand in the middle of that ring of redwoods. Say a word of thanks for the people whose roots intertwine with yours and who nurture and sustain you.

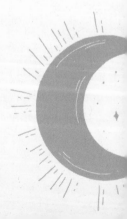

17

CLOUDS

A SAFE LODGING AND A HOLY REST

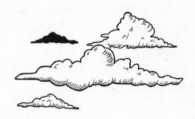

Some of my earliest memories are lying in the backyard behind my house looking up at the clouds while my siblings were at school. The youngest of four, I loved these quiet times on my own. I secretly thought that because I was the one who spent the most time with them and gave them the most attention, the clouds belonged to me—or, at least, that we had a very special relationship, closer than other people had. The clouds would sit still in the sky sometimes, just spending time with me, listening to my thoughts. Other days, they'd give me a quick wave as they moved by, clearly on their way to somewhere important. Storm clouds seemed like they were confiding in me, telling me about why they were in such a bad mood. I loved finding shapes in big, puffy clouds: Rabbits sitting up on their haunches, their ears perked. Cats stretched out on their backs, paws in the air. Angels in flight. I watched and wondered, What stories are the clouds trying to tell?

So when my kindergarten teacher announced that the next day would be "cloud day," my heart raced. She was just back from the main office, where the school's mimeograph machine was housed, with stacks of handouts, the paper still wet and stinking beautifully of that purple ink.

Now I don't remember what hit me—A fever? A cold?—but I had to stay home from school the next day. I missed cloud day. When I returned, evidence of that day's activities was *everywhere*. Ditto sheets of cloud names, shapes, and types. White paper clouds filled with cotton balls and stapled around the edges. My teacher gave me a stack of worksheets in case I wanted to complete them at home. I remember standing by my coat hook at the end of the day paging through the packet. I felt confused and even betrayed. What was the point of doing these *now*? I had missed cloud day. The words on the sheets made no sense: "Match the cloud with its name: cirrus, stratus, cumulus . . ." What were these complicated names for my familiar friends? I tossed the papers, including the baggie of cotton balls, into the trash can.

Years later, I took matters into my own hands and started to bridge that gap in my knowledge, learning the basic names and types. Clouds still capture my attention and my imagination like they did when I was so young. So in case *you* missed cloud day in kindergarten, let's review the basics.

First, you know that clouds are masses of water drops or ice crystals suspended in the earth's atmosphere and that they contain particles of dust, salt, and dirt. When water evaporates from the ground, putting water vapor into the air, it condenses in cooler air, into liquid form, to make clouds.

Temperature, wind, and other factors cause different clouds to form; basically, types of clouds are known by what they look like (cirrus, cumulus, and stratus) and how high up they are (high, midlevel, or low) in our atmosphere. In terms of their appearance, cirrus clouds are thin and wispy, cumulus clouds tend to be big and fluffy, and stratus clouds look like sheets or layers.

The Latin word *cirro* means "curl of hair," and high-level, cirro-form clouds, composed of ice crystals, are the white clouds found at or above about twenty thousand feet. Winds rip these icy clouds into shreds, giving them their feathery appearance. Cirrus, cirrostratus, and cirrocumulus are varieties of high-level clouds.

"Midlevel clouds," with the prefix *alto*, are found between 6,500 and 20,000 feet and are formed mostly of water droplets; when it's cold enough, though, they can be made up of ice crystals. They're normally gray; puffy altocumulus and layered-looking altostratus are two types of midlevel clouds.

By the way, it's nearly impossible to describe cumulus clouds (gray altocumulus or white cumulus) without invoking cotton balls—and equally hard to teach kindergarten students about them without using them in a class project. Yet although they look so light and fluffy, the average cumulus can weigh more than a million pounds.

Low-level clouds, closest to the earth's surface, are found below 6,500 feet; gray, stratus clouds are low-level clouds. Nimbostratus clouds produce falling rain or snow. *Nimbus* is from the Latin, meaning "rain." Low-level clouds fall into four divisions: cumulus, stratus, cumulonimbus, and stratocumulus—the last of which are patchy, gray, and white and resemble a honeycomb.

Like so much in nature, clouds can be much more complex and wayward than simple classifications make them seem. There are many rare and wonderful clouds that don't show up in a classroom introduction. For instance, the Kelvin-Helmholtz cloud looks like a stencil of breaking ocean waves. These are formed when, according to nephologists (meteorologists who specialize in clouds), there's a "velocity difference across the interface between two fluids," like when wind blows over water. These perfect swirls, it's thought, inspired Van Gogh's sky in *The Starry Night*. There are lenticularis clouds, so named because they look like lentils but with an appearance that looks more to most people, including me, like flying saucers. Nacreous clouds, also called "mother-of-pearl" clouds, make the sky look like the brilliant inside of a shell. And there are countless others.

Our companions day and night, clouds are our protectors. They shield us from the sun's glare. They shower us with snow and rain. They blanket us at night. And they spread across the sky in beautiful colors, pictures, and designs, inviting our imaginations to rise and meet them.

◆

Read this prayer from the Book of Common Prayer: "O Lord, support us all the day long, until the shadows lengthen, and the evening comes, and the busy world is hushed, and the fever of life is over, and our work is done. Then in thy mercy, grant us a safe lodging, and a holy rest, and peace at the last. Amen.*"*

◆

In the biblical book of Exodus, a pillar of cloud led the Israelites out of Egypt; it was a manifestation of the Divine.

Do you ever feel the presence of God when you are looking at clouds?

If you imagine clouds as a manifestation of God, what would such a cloud look like?

A cirrus? Thin, white, and wispy and way far up in the sky?

Or do you picture God as more like a cumulus cloud—like a mass of cotton, forming playful shapes in the sky?

Or might God appear as a low-level stratus or like a layer of fog smeared across the face of the sky?

As you prepare for rest, imagine God as a cloud that is leading you into new places, telling you stories in its shapes, and showering you with healing rain.

Close your eyes and picture a blanket of clouds keeping you safe tonight.

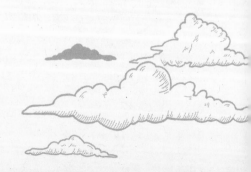

18

CROWN SHYNESS

THE GREAT OPERATIONS OF NATURE

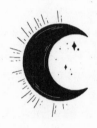

Boundaries exist throughout the natural world: from tiny cell walls to towering mountain ranges to the vast ozone layer that separates our earth's atmosphere from outer space. Maritime boundaries—invisible lines drawn on the face of the sea—divide the ocean, establishing which government controls which part of the expansive whole. Although boundaries can protect and maintain the integrity of a person, place, or thing, they also can be used for harm. When humans construct physical boundaries, we sometimes do so to exclude or marginalize others. The purpose of some boundaries is to maintain distance from the other or to give a sense of security in an insecure, dangerous world. In such borders and boundaries, ideology—just as much as physical bricks, iron, and mortar—is built right in, as we've seen in the construction of the so-called southern border wall between the United States and Mexico, the wall that divided East and West Berlin for almost three decades, the Great Wall of China, and even the creation of placid gated communities. These all speak to and reveal the ideology and convictions of those who manufacture them.

All this to say, boundaries can be *very* complicated things.

William Wordsworth famously advised, "Let Nature be your teacher," and a recent phone call with a friend makes me wonder what nature has to teach us about maintaining healthy boundaries. My friend tells me she's playing emotional tug-of-war with her mother, who is in her seventies. My friend is a gifted singer and has been doing weekly livestream concerts for the past couple of years. It's gone well—the virtual concerts are a reliable source of income, and she has grown her audience. But my friend's mom was the quintessential "stage mother" over the years, and she has recently fallen back into that kind of behavior. Even though her daughter is a middle-aged professional now, the mother frequently posts critiques and compliments in the online comments, during and after the concerts, every week. She insists that her daughter sing some of *her* favorite songs, ones my friend wrote and sang in her youth but no longer performs.

"It's pretty over the top," my friend says, confessing to a tangled mix of feelings: love, guilt, tenderness, embarrassment. She's also experiencing the newly awakened ache of childhood wounds and memories of feeling smothered. She needs *space*, she tells me. She hates the idea of being in conflict with her mother at this point in their lives, but she knows she needs to set better boundaries. And she doesn't want to create a boundary that causes harm or damages her relationship with her mother. It's complicated.

I think of the gentleness of one particular boundary in nature, the phenomenon known as crown shyness. Also called "canopy disengagement" or "intercrown spacing," crown shyness refers to the mysterious spaces—gaps like channels—that exist between neighboring trees in the forest canopy and somehow prevent branches from touching. Certain trees seem to live together as polite neighbors, respecting the invisible boundaries of personal space between them, never allowing their branches to overlap. The branches are alive and thriving and sometimes even waving in the breeze, but given the spaced-apart pattern of their growth, they manage not to touch or cast shade on each other.

You may have seen photographs of trees exhibiting crown shyness or may have even looked up in a forest and seen a gorgeous pattern of gaps between the branches that allows the light to show through. It's like looking out from a plane window and seeing the way meandering rivers cut through the land below; crown shyness in the forest canopy creates rivers in the sky. How and why do trees maintain those boundaries? Like so much in the natural world, we aren't completely sure, but we relish the beauty of this phenomenon, the mosaics those treetops create.

Australian botanist Maxwell Jacobs coined the term *crown shyness* after observing it in eucalyptus trees. Not all trees exhibit it, but crown shyness can also be seen in some oak and pine species, among others. It's most often seen when trees of the same species are growing together and often in trees of similar ages. In the century since Jacobs first discovered this spectacle, there's still not a definitive answer for why it happens. There are, however, a few theories. Jacobs's friction hypothesis is the idea that when the wind blows, the ends of the branches of neighboring trees knock together and are damaged and broken off, causing those gaps. He believed these abrasions hinder the growth of the branches, resulting in trees not touching their nearest neighbors.

Crown shyness is likely the result of many factors, and today, many botanists think that one reason is that trees send messages to each other by releasing "allelochemicals." As mentioned in our exploration of ginkgos, trees can defend themselves from the attack of insects by releasing these negative chemicals. They also release chemicals to signal to other trees, plants, insects, and animals when they want more space or a larger share of nutrients or sunlight.

Trees communicate with each other by sending messages in various ways, not only through their roots and mycorrhizal networks. Via the pores in their leaves and stems, they send signals to the ground or plants below by means of the wind or rain. Messages are also sent into the earth when trees die and their organic matter decomposes; dying trees send carbon and nutrients to nearby trees that are in need. Some trees also release toxic chemicals into the soil around themselves to keep other plants from growing nearby, thus maintaining physical distance from others to reduce the need to compete for resources. Others, for protection, release allelochemicals and send them into their leaves to ward off creatures that would nibble on them—from tiny bugs to animals like giraffes.

A third explanation of crown shyness is that trees and other plants possess light sensors in their leaves known as phytochrome photoreceptors, which allow them to detect light and shade and, therefore, the proximity of other individual plants. When another tree's branches begin to block out the sun, the tree becomes aware of being shaded and then promotes upward, rather than outward, growth.

A benefit of trees maintaining healthy boundaries includes having better access to light, which is essential for photosynthesis, the key to their very survival. It also helps them avoid damage to their branches in the wind and actually protects them from disease. Keeping that space between them—we might think of it as social distancing by trees—prevents the easy movement of the infections or insects that might transfer from one tree to the next. By maintaining boundaries, these trees can better share resources available to them. They can stay healthier. They can grow and thrive.

That doesn't seem so very different from what benefits us human organisms. Good boundaries give us more room for the light to shine through.

◆

Willa Cather is one of my favorite novelists. Her novel O Pioneers!, *published in 1913, is the first of her Great Plains trilogy, followed by* The Song of the Lark *and* My Ántonia. *After its publication, Cather reportedly said that rather than creating a fiction, she had recaptured her memories of "people and places I'd forgotten." Cather wrote many more books and was awarded the Pulitzer Prize for* One of Ours, *a novel set during World War I. Many of her major characters are immigrants; one preeminent scholar claimed that Cather was "the first to give immigrants heroic stature in serious American literature."*

Early on in O Pioneers!, *Alexandra, the protagonist—a child of immigrants and an amazingly resilient person who manages* to thrive in the story despite facing incredible obstacles—looks up at the night sky in wonder.

Read this paragraph from the novel:

Alexandra drew her shawl closer about her and stood leaning against the frame of the mill, looking at the stars which glittered so keenly through the frosty autumn air. She always loved to watch them, to think of their vastness and distance, and of their ordered march. It fortified her to reflect upon the great operations of nature, and when she thought of the law that lay behind them, she felt a sense of personal security. That night she had a new consciousness of the country, felt almost a new relation to it. . . . She had never known before how much the country meant to her. The chirping of the insects down in the long grass had been like the sweetest music. She had felt as if her heart were hiding down there, somewhere, with the quail and the plover and all the little wild things that crooned or buzzed in the sun. Under the long shaggy ridges, she felt the future stirring.

◆

Tonight, as you move toward sleep, imagine looking up at the crowns of trees and seeing a display of crown shyness. Visualize the kind of mosaic the branches and leaves and patches of sky *create. Feel the sunlight coming through the gaps between the tree branches, touching your face.*

Now look inward and take a moment to center yourself, quieting your mind, breathing with intention. Extend loving-kindness toward yourself. Do you need to give yourself permission to be more comfortable and to shine more brightly? Do you need to allow distance between yourself and someone who is keeping you in the shade or seems to absorb too large a share of the nutrients that help you thrive?

Look with compassion on that person, and perhaps imagine maintaining a safe distance between you, giving you a little buffer.

Silently repeat a mantra in your mind:

I am safe.

I am secure.

I am protected.

I have space.

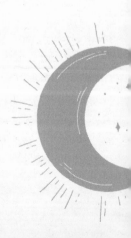

19
PACAYA VOLCANO

WHAT IS FAR OFF AND WHAT IS NEAR

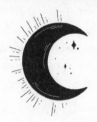

My youngest child, Mia, was born in Guatemala; we adopted her when she was a toddler. On Christmas Eve when Mia was thirteen, my husband and I and our four kids flew from Chicago to Guatemala City to meet her birth family—her birth parents and several of her full biological siblings. The story of that reunion could fill a book; it was a meaningful time, simmering with love and heightened emotion.

In the days leading up to meeting the family, all of us in our individual ways felt expectant and nervous. We were gentle with each other, especially with Mia, as we moved through the week, advancing toward the day when we'd meet her relatives.

We busied ourselves with sightseeing and spent one day at Lake Atitlán, a deep lake surrounded by three cone-shaped volcanoes—Atitlán, Tolimán, and San Pedro—that reflect on its surface. It's hard to describe the stunning beauty of Lake Atitlán without sounding like you're exaggerating. Even John Lloyd Stephens, an American explorer, writer, and diplomat in the early nineteenth century, was in awe of its beauty. And Stephens had been around. Like the Rick Steves of his day, Stephens was a popular travel writer who wrote about his journeys to places like Egypt, Russia, Greece, and yes, Central America. One of his great admirers was Edgar Allan Poe, who reviewed Stephens's travel books in magazines. The Guatemalan poet David Vela described the lake in his poem "Atitlán: Letania en azul cambiante" (in English, "Atitlán: Litany in Changing Blue"), imagining that the lake is where God "made a hole with his finger and filled it with His thought."

In *Incidents of Travel in Central America, Chiapas, and Yucatan*, published in 1848, Stephens describes seeing Lake Atitlán for the first time. He writes, "From a height of three or four thousand feet we looked down upon a surface shining like a sheet of molten silver, enclosed by rocks and mountains of every form, some barren, and some covered with verdure, rising from five hundred to five thousand feet in height." He then said it was "the most magnificent spectacle" he had ever seen. Lake Atitlán is, indeed, magnificent. But the otherworldly scene we'd experience the next day would take me even more by surprise.

On the final day of sightseeing, we visited Pacaya, one of Guatemala's most active volcanoes. Notwithstanding the three-mile climb of eight thousand feet to the top, the tour company managers promised it was an "easy" hike. The easiest, they said, of all the volcanoes in the country.

The night before the hike, I skim through our guidebook, reading to the family about the volcano. We learn that Pacaya first erupted about twenty-three thousand years ago and has erupted dozens of times since the Spanish first invaded Guatemala in 1523. That invasion was prolonged: Mayan kingdoms resisted colonization and were only defeated after about two hundred years. Through it all, Pacaya watched, waited, and blazed. Its activity is mostly what volcanologists term *Strombolian*, meaning it erupts in relatively small blasts. "Peléan" eruptions, by contrast, are more explosive and destructive, quickly pouring thick lava down into surrounding valleys. Volcanoes are classified either by their shapes (including ring, cone, and shield) or by their eruptive behavior. Eruptions (Strombolian, Peléan, Hawaiian) are named after famous volcanoes that erupt in similar ways.

All the talk about eruptions, of course, sparks conversations about how wise it is that we're climbing this volcano in the morning. I assure the kids that we'll be safe—and hope that's true.

The next morning, at the base of the mountain, we meet our guide, Freddie. He tells us that the view from the top, of the surrounding valleys and neighboring volcano Fuego, will be worth any "discomfort" we might experience while making the hike. (*Discomfort?*) My husband and I buy rough-hewn walking sticks from the local children who hover at the mouth of the trail. Freddie nods approvingly and buys one too.

And then we're off. The rocky path starts out innocently enough, gently winding up the mountain. But then the incline gets sharper. The path is soft and uneven, and our feet shift under us; it feels like we are walking uphill in deep sand. My husband and I move ever more slowly and deliberately, step by step by step by step. Our children race ahead, look back at us, and laugh at our slow, methodical pace. I'm too focused on putting one foot in front of the other even to mind. Freddie sportily loops back and forth between us, sometimes stopping up ahead until we catch up to him.

"Oh, they're laughing now," he says. "But they'll feel this tomorrow. You're actually doing it properly." Done properly or not, the climb up Pacaya is the most challenging physical feat I've ever attempted. After a few thousand feet, my body begins protesting the lack of oxygen. I'm short of breath, and sweat pours down my back in the humidity. To add insult to injury, locals on horseback keep circling up and down the trail, approaching the hikers who look most winded—in our group, that's me. "Taxi?" they call, patting their horses on the rump. "Taxi, Lady? Taxi?"

I wave them off, irritated to be forced to expend even an ounce of energy to do so. I am determined to make this hike on my own. My husband and I frequently stop, sip water, and look out over the valleys below and the volcanoes opposite us. At one point, full of insecurity and short of breath, I squawk out to him, using as few syllables as possible, "You going slow for me?"

David shakes his head and says, "No. This is good."

We stand, bent at the waists, and take deep breaths. A huge lava field, evidence of an eruption a few years before, stains a wide swath of the valley below. It's like part of the landscape is blanketed in inky black snow.

After almost two hours, we approach the summit, and the landscape abruptly changes. Instead of the dark, rocky soil under our feet and scrubby trees and plants waving in the breeze, we face a landscape of dried, black lava hills and fields as far as we can see. The top of the volcano is shrouded in clouds, making it all the more otherworldly. I turn around and look back over the valley and at neighboring volcano Fuego. Dark smoke pours from its top. Freddie points out Lake Atitlán, shimmering like a mirror in the distance. Facing the landscape of lava and ash, we move forward. It's like being on another planet. "Welcome to Mordor!" my son calls, and we all laugh.

Stephens wrote about climbing a volcano in Guatemala as well, calling this part of the mountain a "frightful bed." "The lava lay in rolls as irregular as the waves of the sea, sharp, rough, and with huge chasms difficult for us and dangerous for the horses," he wrote. "When we reached the top both my horse and I were almost exhausted."

We continue our climb, now on the lava field, going farther and farther up. Rounding a corner and then descending, we now see only black lava. No valley. No Fuego. No plants or trees. No Lake Atitlán. We can't even see the sky anymore, as we're shrouded in fog. Freddie jogs ahead, motioning us to stop at a level spot in the lava field. He pours a few drops of water into a "hot spot," or crack in the dried lava, and it hisses and steams. Then he unloads his backpack, distributing sandwiches and water bottles. After the seven of us eat lunch at this most unlikely picnic spot, Freddie pulls a bag of marshmallows from his pack. He gives us sticks and shows us where we can toast them, over the hot spots, just a few feet from where we've eaten lunch.

Before we start back down the mountain again, I pick up a few small rocks and then let them drop lightly to the ground. They have very little weight to them; they're porous pumice, formed when hot gases burst out of the rocks and the lava here cooled. I glance over at my daughters. Both girls are holding up toasted marshmallows, laughing and taking a selfie.

I think about the journey we will make tomorrow to meet my daughter's birth family for the first time. I wonder what feelings are hidden under the surface in her right now, simmering, ablaze, but just out of sight.

◆

Read this prayer from the Episcopal Church's Book of Occasional Services:

> *Holy God, your mercy is over all your works, and in the web of life each creature has its role and place. We praise you for ocelot and owl, cactus and kelp, lichen and whale; we honor you for whirlwind and lava, tide and topsoil, cliff and marsh. Give us hearts and minds eager to care for your planet, humility to recognize all creatures as your beloved ones, justice to share the resources of the earth with all its inhabitants, and love not limited by our ignorance. This we pray in the name of Jesus, who unifies what is far off and what is near, and in whom, by grace and the working of your Holy Spirit, all things hold together.* Amen.

◆

Tonight, as you move toward sleep, practice a four-element meditation to become aware of your senses, right here and right now.

The elements are earth, air, water, *and* fire, *and four-element meditations have been practiced for thousands of years by Buddhists, Christian mystics, and others.*

Take a few slow in and out breaths.

Speak the words earth, air, water, *and* fire *silently in your mind.*

Start with the element earth.

Think of your body with kindness. It grounds you, contains you, allows you to move and to touch others.

Focus on the palms of your hands for a moment: What did they hold today? What doors did they open? Whom did they touch? What have they served or given others?

Relax for a few minutes, and let your body sit or lie heavily right where you are.

Earth.

Move on to air.

Notice the air as you slowly breathe in and out. Imagine your lungs inflating as you inhale and then deflating as you breathe out; it's a calm and gentle exchange.

All living things breathe: trees and flowers, birds and sea creatures. Like you, they breathe.

Imagine your lungs inside you, each inhale gathering in and each exhale releasing out.

What do you want to inhale?

What do you want to release?

Breath centers us.
Take a few slow breaths, in and out.
Air.

Move on to water.
Do you feel the water that flows in your own body? In the basal tears that lubricate your eyes? The water in your mouth? About 70 percent of the human body is made up of water; about 70 percent of the earth is covered in it.
Water sustains us.
Water cleanses us.
Water flows.
What flows in you, *right now?*
Water.

Last, move on to fire.
The sun is a ball of fire in the sky. It warms us. It shines its light so we can live. A furnace, a bonfire, and even one candle's flame imitate the sun, radiating heat and light. Your body is a furnace, too, turning fuel into heat and the light you bring into other people's lives.
Imagine lava, deep in the earth, boiling.
Where is the heat in you?
What fuels you?
What warms you?
Fire.

20
THE MOON

HOW IT MOVES IN SILENCE

Last winter, my friend Kathy and I spent a long weekend together in Colorado. While I've never even put on a pair of skis, Kathy is an accomplished downhill skier. I spent the days in our hotel room writing and looking out onto the snowy landscape while she was out on the mountain. I was glad for the change of scenery and for the opportunity for focused time to work. Most of all, I was grateful for the late afternoons and evenings with my friend at the end of each day, sitting in the cozy lodge common area reading, eating dinner, and people watching by the fire.

Every night of our stay, the lounge would fill with the same small cast of characters. One group of eight—adult siblings, their partners, and their parents—often arrived right after we did. They had a child with them, a young boy named Tristan. I know his name because over the course of every meal, they repeated it about one hundred times. Tristan was two or three years old and, like most kids that age, didn't like to sit still. His family would tell him to sit down in his chair, and he'd get restless, bouncing up and down on his knees or sliding his little body onto the floor under the table. ("Tristan! Sit up!") Tristan also didn't much like to eat, so one of the family members would constantly be working to distract him and slip a forkful of pasta or vegetables into his mouth. ("Tristan! Just one bite!")

They worked hard, this family, managing Tristan. One uncle did magic tricks. "Look, Tristan, look!" He'd tear a piece of paper, hold it up, and then—poof—make it disappear. It wasn't long, though, before Tristan was on the move again, and another adult at the table would step up to help. Grandpa would turn the pepper mill into a rocket, or Tristan's mother would draw elaborate tracks on the paper tablecloth, moving Tristan's toy cars around plates and forks and the bread basket. Night after night, we watched as Tristan's family calmed him down by distracting him and appealing to his sense of wonder. It would usually work . . . for a few minutes, anyway.

The last night we were there, this family arrived at the lounge later than they usually did, taking up the long table between where Kathy and I sat and the fire. It was already dark outside, and Tristan looked tired, his face flushed. The service was slower at this later hour, and Tristan *really* didn't want to be in his booster chair. He squirmed and whined and kept trying to slide under the table, but his mother would catch him by the arm and lift him back into place. After a short while, Tristan began to moan and cry.

Just then one of the aunts stood from the table and went around to Tristan's chair. She picked him up, gave him a hug, and then set him on her hip. He stopped crying. Squeezing past Kathy and me, she stood at the window with Tristan. Snow was falling, backlit by a floodlight on the balcony outside. The flakes were big. They looked, somehow, like they were spinning wheels as they fell. A full moon shone over the hills behind the lodge; it was a huge glowing disk of silver, its craters clearer and more visible than I think I've ever seen them.

"Look, Tristan," his aunt said, still holding him gently. "Look up at the moon."

Tristan let his head drop on her shoulder, and then he slowly raised one arm and pointed out the window. "Moon," he said, breathing the word out like a sigh. It seemed like everyone in the room relaxed a bit; we all sat in companionable silence for a while.

We know a lot about the moon, the earth's closest neighbor, but astronomers say it still holds many secrets. We know that ours is one of the largest moons in the solar system but smaller than all of the planets. We believe it was formed about four and a half billion years ago, when the earth, too, was forming. Most scientists agree that a large object collided with the earth at that point, sending a massive amount of debris and magma into space that fell into orbit around the earth and, eventually, combined to form our moon. Composed of rock with a small iron core, the moon's surface is cratered after being battered by asteroids for millions of years. It once had volcanic activity, too, and the cooled lava flows formed the "seas" on the moon's surface. We know now, too, that there is water on the moon. The water may be from its interior, brought to the surface by past volcanic eruptions, or left over from the comets and asteroids—which contain ice—that hit the moon's surface.

From earth, we only see one side of the moon because it's "tidally locked" with the earth, thanks to the earth's gravitational pull. It takes the moon about the same time to rotate on its axis as it takes to orbit once around the earth, so we only ever see its face—and not the so-called dark side of the moon.

We also perceive the moon to be much bigger than it is. That is, although it's four hundred times smaller than our sun, the moon is also four hundred times *closer* to us, so we think of the sun and the moon as the same size. Also, although it appears from earth to be utterly placid and still, there are frequent moonquakes caused by forces including thermal expansion and the impact of meteorites hitting its surface.

That night at the ski lodge, when Tristan's aunt brought him back to the table and lifted him back into his seat, he was strangely calm. Perhaps it was because his meal had finally come and he was hungry enough to eat it. Maybe it was getting near his bedtime. Or maybe the full moon had cast its spell on him, bathing him in awe.

I've tried to make the case for awe in this book, claiming that experiencing wonder and awe is beneficial for a person's mental and physical health. But honestly, wonder is important not just for our own individual sense of well-being; experiencing awe is good for our world. When we experience it, we feel more connected with others. We are more likely to engage in helping behaviors such as donating time, money, or material things to people in need or otherwise giving of ourselves to others. Awe helps us loosen our grip on our privilege, opening our hands to those who don't have access to the advantages that some of us have had.

Like people who have traveled to space and who have been fortunate enough to experience the overview effect, we can allow awe to make us feel less self-interested and less self-important. We can see ourselves as interrelated parts of all of nature and humankind.

This, from an article called "The Proximal Experience of Awe," is a good summary: "People feel awe in response to a variety of experiences—viewing a beautiful sunset across a panoramic landscape, witnessing the birth of a child, or standing in the presence of a powerful, charismatic leader. Our work suggests that not only might people feel awe, wonder, and amazement in response to such events, but also gratitude, love, optimism, and compassion—feelings that may elicit, and be strengthened by, a renewed perspective on oneself and a stronger feeling of connection with others."

Chances are good that no one goes to such great lengths to surprise, calm, or delight you like Tristan's family did for him at the lodge every night. Still, you can intentionally choose—for your own sense of well-being and for the well-being of this world we share—to practice awe.

If you're ever wondering how to do it, take yourself back, in your imagination, to your childhood. Do you remember the sense of wonder that came naturally to you then? Call to mind the way everything from the moon and the stars to an empty cardboard box to a butterfly's wings took you by surprise, held your attention, and fueled your imagination. Maybe you filled your pockets with rocks or pine cones or tiny shells. Maybe you feel a sense of awe now when you see a beautiful work of art in a museum, when you witness a hummingbird hover above a flower, or when a perfect formation of geese flies overhead. Maybe your heart fills with wonder when you remember first seeing your child or grandchild or first meeting the person you now love.

There are many ways to make an intentional practice of experiencing wonder. One is to focus on the moment you're in. Meditation or relaxation practices, like the ones you've sampled while reading this book, help build your "awe muscles." A seeing meditation, for instance, helps us observe something or someone with new eyes. Next time you're with someone you love, try to see them with new eyes. How would a stranger see that face? What would they find beautiful? Maybe you've seen this person a thousand times at every time of day, but try to notice them in a new way. See the hundred universes in them.

Other mindfulness practices you might want to make a regular part of your life include taking deep breaths, practicing loving-kindness toward yourself or others, repeating a mantra or centering phrase, practicing a four-element meditation, doing a smiling practice, or scanning your whole body before going off to sleep. All of these practices can ground us in the moment and open us up to awe. Which of these most resonated with you? Consider making it a nightly habit, a reliable companion for calm at the end of the day.

Lastly, if you are looking to feel more wonder, remember that its close companion is silence. I encourage you to choose silence as you look up and out: maybe into the eyes of someone you love, or at a common dandelion peering up through the cement, or up at the moon, our sun's hand mirror.

Every evening, let silence still you. Draw it around yourself like a protective shawl, and dim the day.

◆

The American naturalist John Burroughs, who said he went to nature to be "soothed and healed," often wrote about the ways he encountered silence in the company of a bird or tree or even in changing weather. He called pine trees "trees of silence," said an owl wing was "shod with silence," and described a coming snowstorm in terms of its silence: "The preparations of a snowstorm are, as a rule, gentle and quiet; a marked hush pervades both the earth and the sky. The movements of the celestial forces are muffled, as if the snow already paved the way of their coming. There is no uproar, no clashing of arms, no blowing of wind trumpets. These soft, feathery, exquisite crystals are formed as if in the silence and privacy of the inner cloud-chambers."

Nature, once again, is our teacher, modeling a practice of silence. And that silence can help us become aware of the presence of the Divine.

◆

Mother Teresa wrote, "We need to find God, and he cannot be found in noise and restlessness. God is the friend of silence.

See how nature—trees, flowers, grass—grows in silence; see the stars, the moon, and the sun, how they move in silence. . . . The essential thing is not what we say but what God says to us and through us."

Tonight, as you close your eyes and move toward sleep, imagine again the "blue marble" image of the earth with its backdrop of outer space. Then pan out in your mind's eye and think of the moon, our earth's closest neighbor, silently watching over you through the night.

Take a few deep breaths: inhale through your nose, and exhale through your mouth.

Practice a loving-kindness meditation for our world.

Repeat these phrases silently:

May the earth be well.

May the earth's people live with ease.

May the earth be protected.

May there be peace.

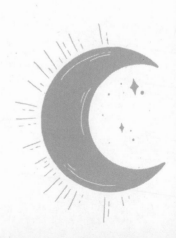

ACKNOWLEDGMENTS

I am hugely thankful for my colleagues and friends at INK: A Creative Collective. Your excellent work and commitment to the common good inspire me. Special thanks to members Lesa Engelthaler, Susy Flory, and Ruth Bell Olsson for reading early drafts of this book and offering guidance and encouragement.

I'm grateful to Mary Andersen, whose stellar work as a research assistant took this content to new and more interesting places.

I'm grateful to ophthalmologist Dr. Stephen Gieser of Wheaton Eye Clinic in Wheaton, Illinois, who generously read and evaluated the content about the human eye.

Thank you, Brian Allain, as ever, for being a trusted colleague and friend. It's an honor to partner with you at Writing for Your Life and Compassionate Christianity.

Thanks to my "Mon Ami Gabi Dinner Club" friends: Glenys Nellist, Caryn Rivadeneira, and Traci Smith for ongoing friendship, laughter, and general spurring on.

My thanks go to Chris Wells—the founding artistic director of thesecretcity.org and a wonderful "creative midwife" for writers—who helped me see my path forward when I was trying to make sense of how to enter into the writing of this book.

Thank you to Rob Feldman for being an early reader and excellent friend (and dependable fellow biophiliac).

Thank you to my yogi, dear friend, and longtime writing partner Jenny Sheffer-Stevens at theregularjenny.com for guidance on framing the relaxation exercises and prompts for sleep.

Valerie Weaver-Zercher, knowing you were waiting in the wings with your sharp intelligence and great sensitivity (and proverbial red pen) made writing this book in this most unusual and distracting time bearable. I received all of your suggestions, edits, and critiques with gratitude.

To my friends Andrea, Cathleen, Jenny, Kathy, and Keiko—even from afar and mostly via text this year, your friendship has sustained me and bolstered me as a writer as it has over so many years.

Thank you to my pandemic bubble mates, lifelines, and walking companions (a.k.a. my husband and children): I couldn't love you more. Last, and never least, David, you're my finest friend. I'm so very fortunate to spend my days and to build my life with you.

A PRAYER

Keep watch, dear Lord, with those who work, or watch, or weep this night, and give your angels charge over those who sleep. Tend the sick, Lord Christ; give rest to the weary, bless the dying, soothe the suffering, pity the afflicted, shield the joyous; and all for your love's sake.
Amen.

—Book of Common Prayer, 124

NOTES

INTRODUCTION

3 **"It would be bizarre"**: Arwa Mahdawi, "We Live in an Age of Anxiety—and We Can't Blame It All on Trump," *Guardian*, August 7, 2018, https://tinyurl.com/ydcuw8cx.

5 **"studies the psychology"**: University of California, Berkeley, Greater Good Science Center (website), accessed April 16, 2020, https://ggsc.berkeley.edu/.

5 **"Awe happens when you"**: Jeremy Adam Smith, "The Benefits of Feeling Awe," *Greater Good Magazine*, May 30, 2016, https://tinyurl.com/y4x9vjw5.

6 **"visual valium"**: Eva M. Selhub and Alan C. Logan, *Your Brain on Nature: The Science of Nature's Influence on Your Health, Happiness and Vitality* (Somerset, NJ: Wiley, 2012), 15–16.

6 **"Additionally, one of Anderson's studies"**: Yasmin Anwar, "Nature Is Proving to Be Awesome Medicine for PTSD," *Berkeley News*, July 12, 2018, https://tinyurl.com/y5kddoz7.

6 **"And, yes, it has"**: Melanie Rudd, Kathleen D. Vohs, and Jennifer Aaker, "Awe Expands People's Perception of Time, Alters Decision Making, and Enhances Well-Being," *Psychological Science* 23, no. 10 (2012): 1130–36.

6 **"In a study published":** Christopher Bergland, "Awe Engages Your Vagus Nerve and Can Combat Narcissism," *Psychology Today*, May 26, 2017, https://tinyurl.com/y6oqtv5b.

9 **"If you look at a thing":** G. K. Chesterton, *The Napoleon of Notting Hill* (New York: William Clowes and Sons, 1904), 5.

10 **"the passionate love":** Erich Fromm, *The Anatomy of Human Destructiveness* (New York: Holt Paperbacks, 1988), 406.

10 **"Whenever there's a crisis":** Rebecca Mead, "The Therapeutic Power of Gardening," *New Yorker*, August 24, 2020, 22.

12 **"Leap and the net":** John Burroughs, *Time and Change*, vol. 13, *The Gospel of Nature* (Boston, 1912; Project Gutenberg, 2004), https://tinyurl.com/yx7t7wr3.

CHAPTER 1

18 **"The only true voyage":** Marcel Proust, *The Captive and the Fugitive*, vol. 5, *In Search of Lost Time* (New York: Modern Library, 1999), 343.

19 **"Man may either blush":** Sebastiaan Mathôt and Stefan Van der Stigchel, "New Light on the Mind's Eye: The Pupillary Light Response as Active Vision," *Current Directions in Psychological Science* 24, no. 5 (2015): 374–78, https://doi.org/10.1177/0963721415593725.

20 **"A university research study":** Aimee I. McKinnon, Nicola S. Gray, and Robert J. Snowden, "Enhanced Emotional Response to Both Negative and Positive Images in Post-Traumatic Stress Disorder: Evidence from Pupillometry," *Biological Psychology* 154 (July 2020): 107922, https://doi.org/10.1016/j.biopsycho.2020.107922.

20 **"In the 1980s":** Olga Khazan, "Can Eye Movement Work like Therapy? A Controversial Treatment Shows Promise, Especially for Victims of Trauma," *Atlantic*, July 27, 2015.

20 **"bringing distressing trauma-related images":** Ramon Landin-Romero et al., "How Does Eye Movement Desensitization and Reprocessing Therapy Work? A Systematic Review on Suggested Mechanisms of Action," *Frontiers in Psychology* 9 (August 13, 2018), https://doi.org/10.3389/fpsyg.2018.01395.

21 **"In their book *Burnout*":** Emily Nagoski and Amelia Nagoski, *Burnout: The Secret to Unlocking the Stress Cycle* (New York: Random House, 2020), 4.

22 **"Going through that emotion":** Nagoski and Nagoski, 18.

CHAPTER 2

28 **"These traits have led":** Francesca Lionetti et al., "Dandelions, Tulips and Orchids: Evidence for the Existence of Low-Sensitive, Medium-Sensitive and High-Sensitive Individuals," *Translational Psychiatry* 8, no. 24 (2018), https://doi.org/10.1038/s41398-017-0090-6.

29 **"incarnation of God":** R. W. Emerson, *Nature* (Boston, 1849; Project Gutenberg, 2009), chap. 7, https://tinyurl.com/jfhypcmp.

29 **"The lover of nature":** Emerson, chap. 1.

30 **"The invariable mark":** Emerson, chap. 8.

CHAPTER 3

35 **"We ran from collecting station":** John Steinbeck and E. F. Ricketts, *The Log from the Sea of Cortez* (New York: Penguin, 1986), 71.

35 **"everything as interrelated"**: "Ed Ricketts and the 'Dream' of Cannery Row: The Legacy of Steinbeck's 'Doc' Endures in Monterey," *Morning Edition*, May 7, 2003, https://tinyurl.com/y2ah83vt.

38 **"common to that breeding ground"**: Cara Giaimo, "In the South Pacific, a Humpback Whale Karaoke Lounge," *New York Times*, September 11, 2019, https://tinyurl.com/y6sh5eyu.

38 **"strange and haunting"**: Carl Safina, *Becoming Wild: How Animal Cultures Raise Families, Create Beauty, and Achieve Peace*, ill. ed. (New York: Henry Holt, 2020), 37.

39 **"Instead, they produce sounds"**: Eduardo Mercado III and Stephen Handel, "Understanding the Structure of Humpback Whale Songs," *Journal of the Acoustical Society of America* 132, no. 2947 (2012), https://doi.org/10.1121/1.4757643.

41 **"Most of the feeling"**: Steinbeck and Ricketts, *Sea of Cortez*, 178–79.

CHAPTER 4

46 **"'Twas brillig"**: Lewis Carroll, "Jabberwocky," Wikisource, last modified November 19, 2018, https://en.wikisource.org/wiki/Jabberwocky.

46 **"no one likes"**: Steinbeck and Ricketts, *Sea of Cortez*, 101.

49 **"Just as the roots"**: John Main, *The Inner Christ* (London: Darton, Longman, and Todd, 1982), 336.

CHAPTER 5

58 **"Never heard happier laughter"**: Genevieve Taggard, "Questions," allpoetry.com, accessed February 18, 2021, https://tinyurl.com/ckna9upb.

CHAPTER 6

61 **"ridiculous 80's-themed"**: Joe Rowlett, "Tosanoides aphrodite, a Spectacular and Very Unexpected New Anthias," reefs.com, 2018, https://tinyurl.com/y2aqw2l7.

62 **"While we were collecting"**: Rowlett.

63 **"cluster of rocks"**: Charles Darwin, *The Voyage of the Beagle* (New York: Doubleday/Anchor, 1962), 5.

64 **"We found on St. Paul's"**: Darwin, 6.

64 **"On its discovery"**: Hudson T. Pinheiro, Claudia Rocha, and Luiz A. Rocha, "*Tosanoides aphrodite*, a New Species from Mesophotic Coral Ecosystems of St. Paul's Rocks, Mid Atlantic Ridge," *ZooKeys* 786 (September 25, 2018), https://tinyurl.com/yy3zfst6.

CHAPTER 7

68 **"I have finally discovered"**: "Manganese Violet," Getty Publications, February 9, 2015, https://tinyurl.com/yy2qnt8b.

68 **"Some studies report"**: Ian M. Paul et al., "Effect of Honey, Dextromethorphan, and No Treatment on Nocturnal Cough and Sleep Quality for Coughing Children and Their Parents," *Archives of Pediatrics & Adolescent Medicine* 161, no. 12 (2007): 1140–46, https://doi.org/10.1001/archpedi.161.12.1140.

68 **"Archaeologists who have found"**: Natasha Geiling, "The Science behind Honey's Eternal Shelf Life," *Smithsonian Magazine*, August 22, 2013, https://tinyurl.com/y7gqqec2.

70 **"When the bees"**: Geiling.

72 **"There is no path"**: Antonio Machado, *Poesias Completas* (Ballingslöv, Sweden: Wisehouse/l'Aleph, 2020), 174.

72 **"Last Night as I Was Sleeping":** Antonio Machado, "Last Night as I Was Sleeping," in *Times Alone: Selected Poems of Antonio Machado*, trans. Robert Bly (Middletown, CT: Wesleyan University Press, 1983), 43.

CHAPTER 8

76 **"In the book":** Judd Apatow, *Sick in the Head: Conversations About Life and Comedy* (New York: Random House, 2015), 195–96.

77 **"When in space":** Ian O'Neill, "The Human Brain in Space: Euphoria and the 'Overview Effect' Experienced by Astronauts," Universe Today, May 22, 2008, https://tinyurl.com/y23nt57v.

78 **"The first thing":** Frank White, "The Overview Effect," August 30, 2019, in *Houston We Have a Podcast*, hosted by Gary Jordan, podcast, https://tinyurl.com/y45jhfhn.

79 **"against the backdrop":** White.

80 **"God save us":** Martin, James. *Between Heaven and Mirth: Why Joy, Humor, and Laughter Are at the Heart of the Spiritual Life.* (New York: HarperOne, 2012), 69.

80 **"Nothing move thee":** Carol Cosman, Joan Keefe, and Kathleen Weaver, *The Penguin Book of Women Poets* (London: Penguin, 1978), 119.

CHAPTER 9

85 **"Clerics, bishops, and others":** Wikipedia, s.v. "Santa Cueva de Montserrat," last modified September 11, 2020, https://tinyurl.com/bp3rdwrc.

88 **"Be patient with all"**: Rainer Maria Rilke, *Letters to a Young Poet: With the Letters to Rilke from the "Young Poet"* (New York: W. W. Norton / Liveright, 2020), 22.

88 **"I love my life's dark hours"**: Rainer Maria Rilke, *The Book of Hours* (New York, 1918; Project Gutenberg, 2012), https://tinyurl.com/sh33mzjk.

CHAPTER 10

97 **"Still alive I am"**: Gábor Terebess, ed., "Matsuo Bashō's Haiku Poems in Romanized Japanese with English Translations," terebess.hu, accessed July 13, 2020, https://tinyurl.com/3aafxe4p.

CHAPTER 11

103 **"I couldn't stand the thought"**: Emily Langer, "Lawrence Anthony, South African Conservationist, Dies at 61," *Washington Post*, March 14, 2012, https://tinyurl.com/y3grzq73.

103 **"One of Anthony's sons"**: Marc Bekoff, "Elephants Mourn Loss of Elephant Whisperer Lawrence Anthony," *Psychology Today*, March 7, 2012, https://tinyurl.com/yyd5mhwa.

105 **"True dignity is like"**: Too-qua-stee, "Dignity," Academy of American Poets, November 3, 2019, https://poets.org/poem/dignity.

CHAPTER 12

111 **"because of his profoundly"**: "The Nobel Prize in Literature 1913," nobelprize.org, accessed November 16, 2020, https://tinyurl.com/yxzewnuf.

111 **"Whatever gifts are in my power"**: Rabindranath Tagore, "The Gift," Your Daily Poem, accessed May 10, 2020, https://tinyurl.com/ru9p798b.

112 **"turn into dust"**: Tagore.

CHAPTER 13

116 **"For the first and second grades"**: Benoit B. Mandelbrot, "A Maverick's Apprenticeship," Imperial College Press, 2002, https://tinyurl.com/y3oe628b.

118 **"The lungs share"**: "Fractals in the Body," Fractal Foundation, accessed September 15, 2020, https://fractalfoundation.org/OFC/OFC-1-2.html.

120 **"for the flowing, endless pattern"**: Viola Spolin, *Improvisation for the Theater* (Evanston, IL: Northwestern University Press, 1999), 14.

120 **"Creativity is an attitude"**: Spolin, 286.

121 **"Almighty and everlasting God"**: *Book of Common Prayer of the Episcopal Church* (New York: Seabury, 1979), 827.

CHAPTER 14

125 **"Redwings nest"**: Hal H. Harrison, *A Field Guide to Western Birds' Nests* (New York: Houghton Mifflin Harcourt, 2001), 228.

125 **"Some studies have shown"**: Priyanka Runwal, "When Yellow Warblers Warn of Brood Parasites, Red-Winged Blackbirds Listen," National Audubon Society, April 6, 2020, https://tinyurl.com/y6rm9nzr.

126 **"Chosen family implies"**: Nina Jackson Levin, Shanna K. Kattari, Emily K. Piellusch, and Erica Watson, "'We Just Take Care

of Each Other': Navigating 'Chosen Family' in the Context of Health, Illness, and the Mutual Provision of Care amongst Queer and Transgender Young Adults," *International Journal of Environmental Research and Public Health* 17, no. 7346 (2020), https://doi.org/10.3390/ijerph17197346.

127 **"In each of these cases":** Levin et al.

128 **"Your friend is your needs":** Kahlil Gibran, *The Prophet* (New York, 1923; Project Gutenberg, 2019), 66, https://tinyurl.com/2jk3d58t.

CHAPTER 15

133 **"a lady's scarf":** John Updike, "The Great Scarf of Birds," *New Yorker*, October 27, 1962, https://tinyurl.com/6zmvbmtk.

134 **"About thirty years earlier":** Peter Friederici, "How a Flock of Birds Can Fly and Move Together," National Audubon Society, March–April 2009, https://tinyurl.com/3stvah7m.

134 **"rapid coordinated":** Sara Brin Rosenthal et al., "Revealing the Hidden Networks of Interaction in Mobile Animal Groups Allows Prediction of Complex Behavioral Contagion," *Proceedings of the National Academy of Sciences of the United States of America* 112, no. 15 (2015): 4690–95, https://doi.org/10.1073/pnas.1420068112.

135 **"He says that the Trinity":** Fr. Richard Rohr, "God Is Relationship," Center for Action and Contemplation, May 9, 2019, https://tinyurl.com/4h5r3wnw.

136 **"I can't help imagining":** Rohr.

137 **"all shall be well":** Julian, Anchoress at Norwich, *Revelations of Divine Love* (London, 1901; Project Gutenberg, 2016), 56, https://tinyurl.com/b3p43thf.

137 **"God All-Power":** Mirabai Starr, *The Showings of Julian of Norwich* (Newburyport, MA: Hampton Roads, 2013), 160.

CHAPTER 16

139 **"whoever came up with":** Anne Lamott, *Plan B: Further Thoughts on Faith* (New York: Riverhead, 2006), 296.

142 **"a plethora of positive health benefits":** Margaret M. Hansen, Reo Jones, and Kirsten Tocchini, "Shinrin-Yoku (Forest Bathing) and Nature Therapy: A State-of-the-Art Review," *International Journal of Environmental Research and Public Health* 14, no. 8 (July 28, 2017): 851, https://doi.org/10.3390/ijerph14080851.

143 **"The forest, she reveals":** "Nature's Internet: How Trees Talk to Each Other in a Healthy Forest," TEDxSeattle, talk by Suzanne Simard, February 2, 2017, https://tinyurl.com/yxo5am9u.

143 **"There are three main types":** *Encyclopedia of Energy*, 2004, s.v. "Carbon Sequestration," accessed September 10, 2020, https://tinyurl.com/y3w7hlkx.

145 **"I am not always in sympathy":** Burroughs, *Time and Change*.

145 **"I go to Nature":** Burroughs.

CHAPTER 17

150 **"velocity difference":** "Kelvin-Helmholtz Clouds," University Corporation for Atmospheric Research, accessed August 15, 2020, https://tinyurl.com/y2xsnmz7.

151 **"O Lord, support us":** *Book of Common Prayer*, 833.

CHAPTER 18

154 **"Let nature be"**: William Wordsworth, "The Tables Turned," Poetry Foundation, accessed July 10, 2020, https://tinyurl.com/y6xcywmo.

157 **"Others, for protection"**: James J. Ferguson, Bala Rathinasabapathi, and Carlene A. Chase, "Allelopathy: How Plants Suppress Other Plants," IFAS Extension, University of Florida, March 2013, https://edis.ifas.ufl.edu/pdffiles/HS/HS18600.pdf.

158 **"people and places"**: Wikipedia, s.v. "*O Pioneers!*," last modified January 11, 2021, https://en.wikipedia.org/wiki/O_Pioneers!.

158 **"the first to give immigrants"**: Susan J. Rosowski, *The Voyage Perilous: Willa Cather's Romanticism* (Lincoln: University of Nebraska Press, 1986), 45.

159 **"Alexandra drew her shawl"**: Willa Cather, *O Pioneers!* (New York: Houghton Mifflin, 1913), 27.

CHAPTER 19

162 **"made a hole with his finger"**: David Vela, *Atitlán: Letania en azul cambiante* (Guatemala: BANCAFE, 2004).

162 **"From a height of three"**: John Lloyd Stephens, *Incidents of Travel in Central America, Chiapas, and Yucatan*, vol. 2 (New York: Harper, 1848), 157–58.

163 **"the most magnificent"**: Stephens.

166 **"frightful bed"**: Stephens, 329.

167 **"Holy God, your mercy"**: I received permission to use this prayer from Church Publishing (see note on the copyright page). This is not a published book, per se, but a resource that is downloadable. If you want to learn more, see Episcopal Church Office of Public

Affairs, "New Liturgical Resource: The Book of Occasional Services 2018," Episcopal News Service, April 9, 2019, https://tinyurl.com/3rctwy2x.

CHAPTER 20

176 **"People feel awe":** S. Katherine Nelson-Coffey et al., "The Proximal Experience of Awe," *PLoS ONE* 14, no. 5 (May 23, 2019), https://tinyurl.com/y5lc6byc.

178 **"soothed and healed":** John Burroughs, *The Writings of John Burroughs* (New York: Houghton Mifflin, 1905), 95.

178 **"We need to find God":** Mother Teresa of Calcutta, *A Gift for God*, repr. ed. (New York: HarperOne, 2003), 76.